The Art of Caregiving in Alzheimer's Disease

Eric Pfeiffer, M.D.

The Art of Caregiving in Alzheimer's Disease

How You Can Help
Your Loved One Cope
with a Monster Disease

With a Foreword by Gayle Sierens,
News Anchor, NBC-TV, Tampa, Florida

Published by Lulu Press, Lulu.com

ISBN 978-1-257-76112-8

Eric Pfeiffer, M.D.
3120 W. Hawthorne Road
Tampa, Florida 33611-2901
Telephone: 813-839-5769
E-mail: epfeiffe@health.usf.edu
Website: ericpfeiffermd.com

Praise for "The Art of Caregiving"

"I wished I had had this book available when I was going through caregiving for my mother."

Dolly Williams, former caregiver

"I think every family member with an Alzheimer's patient should read this book before they go and see the doctor with their loved one. In fact, I think they should make this a Medicare benefit for patients with Alzheimer's disease."

Rena Donze, caregiver whose mother has Alzheimer's disease

"It's easy to read and easy to follow. What a great handbook to have if you are going to look after someone with Alzheimer's!"

Naomi Anders, who has several friends with dementia

Contents

Foreword

More than two decades ago I had the distinct pleasure of meeting Dr. Eric Pfeiffer. As a television news reporter and anchor, it was my job to share with our viewers the latest breakthroughs in medicine. Here in Florida, a great deal of that news deals with our aging population, of which I am now a part. I had the good fortune to meet and interview this brilliant man whose passion it is to better the lives of the elderly, and help the rest of us understand what they are facing and in many cases, already dealing with. Little did I know then that I would be one of those people. I am the only child of a mother who is moving into the late stages of Alzheimer's. It's hard to understand that world unless you are in the middle of it. But Dr. Pfeiffer has given us not only a glimpse into that world with his book "The Art of Caregiving in Alzheimer's," he has taken us by the hand and given us a step by step guide of how to walk that path, with courage and armed with information. I am grateful to have this most useful tool as I make my way through this puzzling disease, and I am thankful that Eric Pfeiffer continues his compassionate efforts on behalf of those who have the disease, and those of us who care for our loved ones.

Gayle Sierens, News Anchor, NBC-TV, Tampa, Florida

Introduction

If you are considering becoming a caregiver of someone afflicted with Alzheimer's disease, or if you have been thrust into the role of caregiver to someone with the disease, this book is for you. It is intended as your personal guide to a journey the likes of which you have never before experienced. Even if you have raised children, taught school, supervised employees, or have in other ways taken on responsibility for someone else, becoming an Alzheimer's caregiver will challenge you as well as enrich you in ways you could not possibly imagine. Or, if you have never have been in a position in which you were charged with caring for someone else, you will find that caring for someone with Alzheimer's creates demands and opportunities of an entirely different order of magnitude than anything else you have ever encountered: because *Alzheimer's is a disease like no other*. Its manifestations will change continually and progressively before your very eyes, and before you know it, you too will be changed forever by being a caregiver to someone with this disease. Possibly you will be changed for the better, in ways that I will explain to you throughout the book.

The reason I have written this book is that I have seen this disease at close range in my role as the treating physician for thousands of Alzheimer's patients. In that role I have also had the opportunity of seeing thousands of caregivers deal with the challenge presented by this disease. In doing so I have learned a great deal about caregiving from these same caregivers. I have seen them struggle with increasingly complex issues. I have seen them develop innovative approaches, creative attitudes, and ingenious techniques that allowed them to make a success of their caregiving experience, i.e. they became *consummate* caregivers. In the process they reaped unforeseen rewards, and discovered strengths they never knew they possessed. Some of them have truly become modern-day heroes, as they learned, through trial and error, and from each other, what worked and what didn't work. It is *their* cumulative wisdom and experience that I would like to convey to light your way as you embark on the remarkable journey that lies ahead.

In this book I will also convey to you some of the fundamental knowledge we have today about Alzheimer's disease. It is a *disease of the brain,* not simply a manifestation of aging. To date we do not fully understand the causes of this remarkable disease, but real progress is being made towards this goal, with much more to come in the months and years ahead. Understanding the nature of this disease will help you as you assume your role as a caregiver for someone with Alzheimer's. And it will help you to make a positive difference in the life of your loved one.

Thank you for opening this book and for opening your mind to the suggestions and guidance offered here. You will find information that will not only make you a competent but a *consummate* caregiver to someone with Alzheimer's disease.

Chapter One

What is a Caregiver?

A caregiver is someone who takes care of another person who is either sick or disabled. A caregiver does those things, and only those things, that the sick or disabled person can no longer do independently. In other words, what a caregiver does depends on just what that other person needs to have done for them. And that may depend on the stage or the severity of the illness or disability. In some cases, and at some stages of a disease, it may involve giving only a little bit of help: steadying the person's gait, combing their hair, helping them to get dressed, or helping them to get to the bathroom on time. In other cases it can go much further, to the point, in fact, where the caregiver does virtually *everything* for the other person. So now you are getting the idea what may be involved in being a caregiver to someone with any kind of disease or disability. In this book, however, we are going to talk specifically about what is involved in becoming a caregiver *to* someone with Alzheimer's disease. Here are some of the specifics that apply:

a. Caregivers are the life-line to patients with Alzheimer's disease.

This is no overstatement. Without caregivers, patients with Alzheimer's disease could not find their way to the doctor; they could not accurately provide their own history, neither the history of their illness nor the history of their lives. They could not convey to the doctor the extent of their memory problems, or the behavioral problems that complicate their memory deficits. What caregivers do is vitally important to the patient: it may include preparing meals, taking the patient to the doctor, carrying out the doctor's orders, such as giving the patient their medication. It includes as well providing emotional support, love, and affection. Caregivers also help patients to make decisions or, later on in the disease, when the patient can no longer participate in decision-making, they must make decisions on their patient's behalf. Caregivers serve as advocates for the patient. They become *the guardian angel* of the patient, hovering near-by, preventing the patient from missteps or harm, but only taking over what the patient can no longer do independently, encouraging the patient to exercise all the skills they still possess.

b. Caregivers are vital decision-makers regarding treatment.

Caregivers, almost as much as physicians, are also decision-makers about when Alzheimer's patients begin treatment, and whether they continue on active and effective treatment. For this reason it is critically important for caregivers to understand the nature of the illness and the nature of available treatments, their benefits, limitations, potential side-effects, and the changing pattern of behaviors over the course of the disease. Unless caregivers have realistic expectations about what medications can accomplish they are not in a position to make good decisions on behalf of the patient.

c. Caregivers are the doctors' partners in implementing a treatment program.

Not only do caregivers need to understand the purpose of treatment but they must work with the doctor to observe and report beneficial or adverse changes in the patient's response. They are the ones to refill or renew the patient's prescriptions, and carry out any other instructions given by the doctor. Since Alzheirner's disease can last anywhere from two to twenty-five years, it is clear that doctor and caregiver need to establish a long-term partnership with mutual trust and respect. For this reason I advise that doctor and caregiver spend time with each other on each visit, away from the patient, so that neither the doctor nor the caregiver is constrained from raising issues which could not be comfortably discussed in the presence of the patient.

d. Caregivers assure quality of life for the patient

While doctors can diagnose and make treatment recommendations, the day-to-day quality of life rests largely in the hands of the family caregiver. Their efforts to provide continuity, dignity, pleasure, social interaction, a stable environment, and freedom from unwanted surprises, make a huge difference in the life of an Alzheimer's patient. What the caregiver does determines in large part how patients deal with their fate, resulting in either calm acceptance of the disease or in lashing out against the caregiver and the rest of the world.

Some people are natural-born caregivers. They do all the right things, without instruction. But other caregivers don't know where to start, and may need a lot of help. I am hoping that this book will provide some of the necessary guidance. I want to convey to you all that I know about the illness, about available treatments, and how to manage disruptive behaviors when they occur. At the University of South Florida we have developed a series of caregiver classes to teach family members about the illness, about available treatments, techniques for managing disruptive behaviors, and available community resources such as day care and respite care. These classes also teach how to prepare legally and financially for the caregiver experience, with information about durable family power of attorney, health surrogate instruments, and living wills. In our caregiver classes we use the natural-born caregivers as teachers and models of care provision.

If no such caregiver classes exist in your community you might advocate with your doctor or your memory disorder clinic that they begin such classes. The participants in our caregiver classes have called them true *life-savers!* In the chapters that follow I will try to give you the information and explanations you need to function as an effective caregiver.

e. Caregivers may be at risk of themselves becoming patients

Given the demands and stresses of caregiving, it should not be surprising that some caregivers may become patients themselves, at times succumbing to depression, burnout (sometimes called compassion fatigue), or self-neglect. To minimize the risk of this happening, caregivers need emotional support, recognition, encouragement, suggestions for coping techniques, and information about their role as caregivers. For this reason we recommend that you take a little time at each doctor visit for your loved one to talk about how *you* are faring in your caregiver role.

e. There are distinct stages of caregiving.

As there are distinct stages of Alzheimer's disease, described in detail in subsequent chapters, there are also distinct stages of caregiving. Briefly, they are as follows:

Stage 1: Coping with the initial impact of being told the diagnosis.

Stage 2: Deciding whether you or some other family member will take on the caregiver role.

Stage 3: The long stretch of at-home caregiving.

Stage 4: Considering residential placement.

Stage 5: Caregiving during residential placement of the patient.

Stage 6: Death of the patient, grief, and a sense of relief.

Stage 7: Resuming your life after Alzheimer's — healing and renewal.

As a caregiver, you may need assistance and counseling at each of these stages in order to cope with the changing experience so as not to become a patient yourself. I will try to prepare you for each of these stages, and I will tell you where to get help and support if and when the going gets rough.

Chapter Summary

1. **A caregiver is someone who takes care of another person that is either sick or disabled.**

2. **Caregivers are the life-line to patients with Alzheimer's disease.**

3. **Caregivers are vital decision-makers regarding treatment.**

4. Caregivers are the doctor's partners in implementing a treatment program

5. Caregivers assure quality of life for the patient.

6. Caregivers may be at risk of themselves becoming patients.

7. There are distinct stages of caregiving.

Chapter Two

Why Would You Want to Become A Caregiver?

That is a good question. The only reason you would consider becoming a caregiver is that the other person needs care, and you are the only logical person to provide that care. Why? Because you love them, or because you are committed to them in some profound way, most often through blood or marriage. And what would that mean for you? I mean, don't you have your own life to live? How could you become a full-time caregiver? It would mean giving up a good part of your own life, or taking on this work in addition to whatever you are doing with your own life. Isn't that asking rather a lot? Indeed it is. So why would you want to become a caregiver?

In truth, nobody *wants* to be a caregiver. You only do it because you have caregiving thrust upon you, by fate, or circumstance, or by being who you are or what you are at this time in your life. So how and why is it that you are even considering becoming a caregiver at all, much less, a consummate caregiver?

There is no law that says you have to be the one to become the patient's caregiver. You can decide that it is simply not something you can do or want to do, and then you have to find someone else to take on this task: another relative, a friend, or a paid care manager. But you must decide this fairly early on. The fact that you are reading this book seems to indicate that you have made the decision to take on this role. But remember, it is a choice. You can still change your mind, before it is too late.

I, for my part, am going to try to do everything possible to help you carry out this choice with skill and elegance and yes, even joy. Given that caregiving can be a very demanding and stressful activity, and given that it can go on over extended periods of time, you wouldn't want to take on this kind of responsibility except for someone whom you love or to whom you are deeply committed. So for the most part caregivers will provide care only to someone really close to them: a spouse, a sibling, a parent or an in-law. Occasionally someone will become a caregiver to a really good friend. In any case, a strong commitment to the person for whom you are going to provide care is absolutely necessary.

Why should someone you love need a caregiver?

Why would someone you love need a caregiver? How did they suddenly lose their ability to care for themselves? No, they didn't suddenly become lazy, or take on airs and demand to be treated like a prince or a princess. They were just living their life in all innocence. And then something happened. *They developed Alzheimer's disease.* Well, they could have developed some other problem such as severe arthritis, a stroke with significant residual consequences, or something else. Some of the same principles may also apply to caregiving for other illnesses or disabilities. Here, however, our focus will be on Alzheimer's disease caregiving specifically.

You have to consider becoming a caregiver only because someone close to you --your spouse, your brother or sister, your mother or mother-in-law, rarely even an adult child -- has developed Alzheimer's. And Alzheimer's *demands* caregiving.

Chapter Summary

1. There are good reasons for becoming a caregiver.

2. Nobody really WANTS to become a caregiver.

3. There are good reasons why someone would need a caregiver.

4. Alzheimer's disease *demands* caregiving.

Chapter Three

The Rewards of Caregiving

Before you become too overwhelmed by the idea of being a caregiver, with all that it entails, let me spend just a little time talking about all the rewards of caregiving. There are in fact surprisingly many. In talking about the possible rewards, it may well be that those that I mention first will be the least important to you, and those mentioned later the most important one, or vice versa. You will be able to sort them out, so here goes, in no particular order.

a. What you are doing is an act of love, or of "love made work." Acts of love reward the person giving love at least as much as the person receiving it. Here is a brief illustration of how this works:

> *Jonathan is an eighty-year old caregiver whose wife Mary is now in a nursing home where she has been for the past two years. Every morning he visits the nursing home to have breakfast with her. He continues to do so even though he realizes she no longer knows who he is. One day a friend asked Jonathan why he kept visiting Mary even though she no longer recognized him. Smiling, Jonathan patted his friend on the shoulder and said: "She doesn't know me,* **but I still know her.***" Jonathan's reward was in giving love, not in receiving it.*

b. What you are doing is literally life-saving to the person with Alzheimer's disease. Here is an illustration:

> *Henry and Jane were divorced after some twenty years of marriage when Henry took up with a younger woman. Jane watched from afar and saw Henry's new relationship fall apart. When Henry developed Alzheimer's disease on top of the diabetic condition which he had had for some years, the younger woman was nowhere to be found. As she saw Henry's disease progress to the point where he could no longer care for himself and would need to go to a nursing home, **Jane moved back in with Henry** and cared for him, saving him from an early admission to a nursing home, or from coming to harm in some other way. When asked why she was doing this she just shrugged her shoulders and smiled. Maybe it was her way of getting back at her husband for his unfaithfulness, or maybe it was in honor of the love they had shared for a long time.*

c. You will be challenged like you have never been challenged before, and you will rise to the challenge time and again. You will see yourself grow by leaps and bounds.

d. Your acts of caregiving will tame this disease and lessen its force on your loved one, allowing them to still be more like themselves, in their actions, in their personality, and in their communications with you.

e. As a caregiver, you will meet many other courageous caregivers, and you may form new friendships that will last you the rest of your life. Here is an illustration:

> *Helen, Marion, Martha, and Edith all belonged to the same caregiver support group. Each had a*

*husband with Alzheimer's disease, at differing stages of the disease. Each of the four came from almost totally different backgrounds and would likely never have met each other in the ordinary course of social interactions. But somehow they developed a common bond, called themselves "the gang of four", met outside of the support group with each other, and long after their caregiving days were over, kept up their friendship as each of them went on to experience differing illnesses and other life challenges. Whereas before they were there to support their husbands and each other, now **they were there just to support each other**, an unexpected reward bestowed on them as a result of a common tragic experience.*

f. You will be participating in one of the most heroic battles that science has ever fought with a disease, and someday you may be celebrating, with many others "a world without Alzheimer's." Here is another illustration:

*Anita's mother suffered from Alzheimer's disease. She sought out the best available treatment for her mother, moving her clear across the country so that she could participate in an experimental study with a new medication for the treatment of Alzheimer's. While her mother benefited from the new drug, she nevertheless went on to eventually die from the disease. Grateful for the care provided to her mother, Anita donated a large amount of money to the research center with which she had worked, **establishing one of the first endowed research centers on Alzheimer's disease**. This center went on to discover additional medications and treatment approaches that eased the burden of* *the disease for thousands of other patients in the center's service area as well as throughout the country. Anita had made a real difference in the battle against Alzheimer's disease.*

To be sure, caregiving for someone with Alzheimer's disease is one of the hardest jobs anyone will ever face. Yet caregiving has to be done -- by someone. What I have tried to do in these few remarks is to tell you that if you have chosen to take on this challenge, however much you give to this job, you will be amply and multiply rewarded.

Chapter Summary

1. **Caregiving is an act of love.**

2. **Caregiving is life-saving to the patient with Alzheimer's disease.**

3. **Caregiving will be your greatest challenge in life.**

4. **Caregiving tames Alzheimer's disease.**

5. **As a caregiver you will meet other caregivers.**

6. **You will be making a contribution towards creating A world without Alzheimer's Disease."**

Chapter Four

Alzheimer's: A Disease like No Other

So what is Alzheimer's disease? It is a disease of the brain whose cause is not fully understood. It affects people in their later years, through no fault of their own. It gradually takes over, first a few, then more and more areas of a person's life. It is in fact a disease like no other. It affects nearly six million people in the United States at this time, and that number is going to *double* in the next twenty years. The reason for this is that more and more people live into their seventies, eighties, and nineties, and the prevalence of the disease increases drastically with each advancing decade. Thus, only ten percent of people in their seventies have the disease, but it increases to thirty percent of people in their eighties, and to nearly fifty percent of people in their nineties. Some people have called Alzheimer's a *monster disease*, not only because if affects a huge number of people, but also because of what it does to those affected. It gradually eats away layer after layer of human functioning, starting with memory and decision-making capacity, and continuing to erode deeper and deeper layers of the personality. It attacks language, judgment, ability to communicate, and self-care capacity. Even more vexing than these losses is an accumulation of troublesome behaviors which increase gradually as the disease advances. Effective caregiving is what humanizes this ordeal, both for the patient and the caregiver. Caregiving is what makes it possible to *live with this disease* rather than be overwhelmed by it.

In subsequent chapters I am going to discuss in detail how this disease unfolds, and how caregivers can respond to its many manifestations. I am going to explain how scientific advances and caregiver strategies are moving forward *to tame this disease.* And I am going to be by your side every step of the way as you accompany the person affected by the disease every step of the way.

Alzheimer's disease comes on like rain in the night, imperceptibly at first, until it amounts to a flood that threatens to swallow both you the caregiver and the person affected by Alzheimer's disease. Let me give you a brief illustration of how Alzheimer's disease can sneak up on both patient and caregiver:

> *Jack and Susan were friends of ours, she an accomplished college professor, he a successful publisher. It was a second marriage for each of them. Perhaps this contributed to the fact that both of them were slow to notice that anything was wrong, as each tended to pass off what was happening as just an adjustment to the new relationship. Jack began to forget conversations he had had with Susan, which she wrote off as his simply being overly occupied with his work. Jack began to forget mutually agreed-upon social appointments, and also became less attentive to his personal hygiene. Again, Susan did not want to criticize Jack, as their relationship was still relatively new and she feared offending him. It was finally his children who pulled Susan aside and confronted her with the fact that Jack's forgetfulness and his need for reminders to take a bath or to change clothes, was a significant change in his behavior which they felt needed medical attention. This was hard for Susan to accept, as Jack continued to be charming and socially competent, continued to use his erudite vocabulary, and continued to do the Sunday New York Times crossword puzzle without*

difficulty. But she heeded his children's concern and had Jack evaluated by a neurologist. The neurologist found problems with short term memory, problems with delayed recall of new information, and had an MRI scan of the brain done that showed atrophy in a small portion of the temporal lobe which serves memory. This news was shocking to both Jack and Susan. However, they accepted the doctor's assessment and followed his treatment recommendations. They continued to show their love for each other, and Susan reluctantly came to realize that she would have to become the caregiver to Jack, brilliant though he was. Susan consulted me both as a friend and as an expert on Alzheimer's disease, joined a caregiver support group, learned everything she could about the disease and about caregiving, and cared for Jack, through all the stages of the disease, until he died some seven years later.

It is important to realize that Alzheimer's is a disease, not simply a manifestation of old age. It is a disease in which brain cells die prematurely and progressively, leaving the individual with gradually decreasing abilities in their thinking, feeling and behavior. In the next few chapters I am going to discuss all the stages of Alzheimer's disease, mild, moderate and severe, and provide you with strategies to respond to each of these stages.

However, Alzheimer's disease is not the only memory problem which can crop up in later life. Before going on to describe Alzheimer's disease in detail, let me first discuss some of the less serious memory problems which can also occur as people get older. Then you will be able to see more clearly how Alzheimer's disease fits into the whole spectrum of memory disorders.

Chapter Summary

1. Alzheimer's is a disease of the brain.

2. Alzheimer's disease is huge in terms of numbers of people affected and the impact it has on those affected.

3. Alzheimer's disease "comes on like rain in the night."

Chapter Five

Less Serious Memory Problems

There are at least three types of memory problems that can happen to people as they get into their sixties, seventies and eighties. I will discuss only the two less serious ones in this chapter, i.e. *benign forgetfulness* and *mild cognitive impairment*. The third, *Alzheimer's disease,* will be discussed in the chapters that follow.

Benign forgetfulness

Benign forgetfulness happens to the majority of people over age 65. It is annoying but not serious. Benign forgetfulness is characterized by relatively minor slowing of your memory capacity and manifests itself in a number of little ways such as forgetting where you parked your car, or recognizing someone at a social gathering but being unable to recall their name right then and there. (A little while later the name comes back to you, and you feel somewhat foolish.) Or, it may be a matter of having more difficulty in learning new information: learning how to operate new gadgets or remembering new phone numbers may not be as easy as it was years ago.

With a little extra concentration, these problems can usually be overcome. You may need to write down new information; you may need to make associations between familiar names or words with an unfamiliar word or name you are trying to learn in order to better remember it. You may have to have someone show you more than once how your new iPhone or DVD player works. But you can still learn. You can still remember; you may just have to work at it a little harder. You may need to write yourself more notes, jot down the aisle number where you parked your car, or *always* place your house keys, your purse, or your wallet in exactly the same spot every time you come into the house. The good news about benign forgetfulness is that it doesn't get any worse, and it does not lead to Alzheimer's disease. The bad news is that it doesn't get any better, either. You need to understand it, accept it, and adjust to it in ways like those above.

Mild cognitive impairment

Mild memory impairment, or more formally, *mild cognitive impairment,* is serious, but not fatal. Mild cognitive impairment is characterized by completely forgetting whole sequences of events in which you have actively participated. This can be embarrassing, or worse. For instance:

John, age 70, lived in Florida and regularly went to an annual family reunion in Tennessee. Last year, when he came back, his son-in-law asked him about the reunion. John said he had not attended at all. But his daughter, who also attended, had recorded a videotape of the reunion. When John saw the video, clearly showing him as participating and interacting at the event, he broke into tears. He realized fully for the first time that he had completely forgotten about the event. He also realized the implications of the occurrence: his memory problems were far greater than mere absentmindedness.

What happens in minor cognitive impairment is that the brain participates in the actual experience but no memory trace is laid down. It is somewhat like not pressing the "enter" or the "save" button on your computer. If such a situation occurs more than once or twice, you should undergo a thorough memory evaluation by a specialist in memory disorders, someone beyond your primary care doctor. This could be a psychiatrist, a neurologist, or an internist, but, in any case, it should be a doctor who has a strong interest and extensive experience in memory evaluations. Standard memory tests may need to be performed. In addition, your ability for *delayed recall* of information may need to be tested. Delayed recall, that is, recall of information that had just recently been presented, is one of the earliest signs of mild cognitive impairment.

Further evaluation may require a session with a trained neuropsychologist, an MRI (magnetic resonance imaging), or a PET (positron emission tomography) scan. An MRI is a test that produces an actual image of the brain, and it can pick up early indications of brain cell loss. A PET scan is similar but even more specialized and expensive, and it can pick up changes in brain cell activity or metabolism before there is any loss of brain tissue.

If you or someone close to you is diagnosed with mild cognitive impairment, it can and should be treated by a memory specialist. Medications that have already been approved for the treatment of Alzheimer's disease, such as Aricept, Exelon, or Razadyne, have been shown to be of benefit to persons with minor cognitive impairment as well. While mild cognitive impairment isn't the same thing as Alzheimer's disease, it can progress to Alzheimer's disease if left undiagnosed and untreated.

Chapter Summary

1. **Benign forgetfulness is common in older persons**

2. **Mild cognitive impairment is a more serious memory problem**

3. **And then there is Alzheimer's disease.**

Chapter Six

Understanding Alzheimer's Disease

Alzheimer's disease, on the other hand, is a problem of an entirely different order of magnitude. It is, first of all, a disease of the brain, not merely a manifestation of aging. It is a disease in which brain cells die prematurely and progressively. This leaves an individual with impaired memory function, impaired decision-making ability, and reduced reasoning and learning capacity. It is a very variable disease which can last anywhere from two to more than 20 years, eventually resulting in death, unless the person dies from another illness before then. President Ronald Reagan, for instance, lived with Alzheimer's disease for 17 years.

In some individuals, Alzheimer's is primarily characterized by increasing degrees of memory and intellectual decline. Others with Alzheimer's may also exhibit behavioral problems, which can often be more vexing to the caregiver than memory problems. Behavioral problems can include depression, agitation, irritability, hostility, and even hallucinations and/or delusions. It is one thing to care for a nice little old lady who may be a bit forgetful but who is otherwise pleasant, and quite another to deal with someone who is hostile, suspicious, aggressive, or fears that the caregiver is trying to poison him.

Thus it is not surprising that Alzheimer's disease is sometimes referred to "the big A" by patients and family members. It can indeed be a devastating disorder. Therefore, when it is suspected, it urgently requires prompt diagnosis, followed immediately by treatment in order to preserve memory and intellectual capacity at the highest possible level for as long as possible.

Now let me acquaint you with some of the hallmarks of Alzheimer's disease. I have called them "The Seven Warnings Signs of Alzheimer's Disease," and they have been widely published, by the Suncoast Alzheimer's and Gerontology Center at the University of South Florida and elsewhere. These signs have been helpful in alerting both lay persons and professionals to the fact that a serious memory problem may exist. Here they are:

The Seven Warning Signs of Alzheimer's Disease

1.   Asking the same question over and over again

2.   Repeating the same story, word for word, again and again.

3.   Forgetting how to cook, or how to make repairs, or how to play cards -- activities that were previously done with ease and regularity.

4.   Losing one's ability to pay bills or balance one's checkbook.

5.   Getting lost in familiar surroundings, or misplacing household objects.

6.   Neglecting to bathe, or wearing the same clothes over and over again, while insisting that they have taken a bath or that their clothes are still clean.

7.   Relying on someone else, such as a spouse, to make decisions or answer questions they previously would have handled themselves.

The presence of two or three of these signs should alert you to the fact that a serious problem may exist. Four or five of these signs are definite signs of a major problem. And if all seven of these signs are observed, the person manifesting them almost definitely has Alzheimer's disease or another form of dementia.

Dementia is defined as any memory disorder due to the loss of brain cells. Alzheimer's disease is one of the causes of dementia. Other causes of dementia may include a major stroke, or multiple smaller strokes, traumatic brain injuries, chronic alcoholism, or encephalitis. Dementia can also occur in the late stages of Parkinson's disease or as the result of Lewy Body disease, a variant of Alzheimer's disease. If checking for the seven warning signs of Alzheimer's disease doesn't give you an answer, and you are still concerned about a family member or friend, there is another test available. At Duke University I developed the *Short Portable Mental Status Questionnaire* (See Figure 1) to measure the presence and the degree of memory loss. The questionnaire is usually administered by a doctor, a nurse, or a social worker, but a layperson can do this as well. Accordingly, *you* could ask someone about whose memory you are concerned these questions to determine if they are experiencing significant memory loss. Please note that this is not a self-administered test. It allows the examining person to determine if the person's memory is normal, or whether he or she has mild, moderate, or severe memory loss, according to the scale shown on the next page. However, the test does not allow one to make a definitive diagnosis of Alzheimer's disease, or of any other memory specific disorder for that matter. If there is evidence of significant memory loss, a full medical evaluation should be arranged as soon as possible.

A score of none to two errors usually means normal memory function. A score of three to four errors is indicative of mild memory impairment. Five to seven errors indicate moderate impairment, and a score of eight to ten errors means severe memory impairment. The score only indicates the severity of the impairment. It does not indicate the specific cause of the memory impairment, and therefore cannot be used as a diagnostic tool. You will find a discussion of how Alzheimer's disease *is* diagnosed in Chapter 7.

SPMSQ	**PFEIFFER**
	SHORT PORTABLE MENTAL STATUS QUESTIONNAIRE

INSTRUCTIONS: Ask the subject questions 1-10, record answer, and enter as "1" under appropriate column (correct/error). All responses, to be scored correct, must be given by subject without reference to calendar, newspaper, birth certificate or other memory aid.	Patient Name: Date:

		CORRECT	ERROR
1.	WHAT IS THE DATE TODAY? Month_____ Day_____ Year_____ (Score correct only when the exact month, day and year are given correctly.)		
2.	WHAT DAY OF THE WEEK IS IT? Day_____		
3.	WHAT IS THE NAME OF THIS PLACE? _____ (Score correct if any correct description of the location is given: "My home," accurate name of town, city or name of residence, hospital, or institution (if subject is institutionalized) are all acceptable.)		
4.	WHAT IS YOUR TELEPHONE NUMBER? (If none see 4A below) (Score correct when the correct number can be verified or when subject can repeat the same number at another point in question.) #_____ 4A. WHAT IS YOUR STREET ADDRESS? (Ask only if subject does not have a telephone.) _____		
5.	HOW OLD ARE YOU? AGE:_____ (Score correct when stated age corresponds to date of birth.)		
6.	WHEN WERE YOU BORN? Month_____ Day_____ Year_____ (Score correct only when exact month, date, and year are all given.)		
7.	WHO IS PRESIDENT OF THE UNITED STATES NOW?_____ (Only the last name of the President is required.)		
8.	WHO WAS THE PRESIDENT BEFORE HIM?_____ (Only the last name of the previous President is required.)		
9.	WHAT WAS YOUR MOTHER'S MAIDEN NAME?_____ (Does not need to be verified. Score correct if a female name plus last name other than subject's is given.)		
10.	SUBRACT 3 FROM 20 AND KEEP SUBTRACTING 3 FROM EACH NEW NUMBER ALL THE WAY DOWN. ___ ___ ___ ___ ___ ___ (The entire series must be performed correctly in order to be scored correct. Any error in series or unwillingness to attempt series is scored as incorrect.)		

	TOTAL NUMBER OF ERRORS	
***ADJUSTMENT FACTOR**		
A)	SUBTRACT 1 FROM ERROR SCORE IF SUBJECT HAS HAD ONLY A GRADE SCHOOL EDUCATION	-
B)	ADD 1 TO ERROR SCORE IF SUBJECT HAS HAD EDUCATION BEYOND HIGH SCHOOL	+
	TOTAL ADJUSTED ERRORS	

SCORING KEY: 0-2 errors = intellectually intact; 3-4 errors = mildly impaired;
5-7 errors = moderately impaired; 8-10 errors = severely impaired.

INFORMATION OBTAINED BY:	DATE:

You Are Beginning to Suspect that it Might Be Alzheimer's Disease.

At the present time nearly everyone is aware to a greater or lesser degree of the possibility of Alzheimer's disease. We joke about it when we have forgotten a name or an event or where we parked out car, saying "it must be my Alzheimer's kicking in." (By the way, Pfeiffer's law says that people only joke about those things that they are most serious about.) But Alzheimer's is no joking matter. If someone close to us repeatedly fails to remember important information and that fact constitutes a change from their previous behavior, we have every reason to be suspicious that something serious is going on. If you observe one or two or even three of the warning signs of Alzheimer's disease I have just discussed, your concerns may be heightened. So you will need to continue your observations. Remain watchful for other signs of a faulty memory, of a lack of attention, or of an inability to complete a task the loved one has begun. You will want to believe that it's not Alzheimer's. But that would be denial. And denial has its useful aspect: it protects us from pain or anxiety. Its downside is that it leads us to ignore a problem that should not be ignored.

Now you might think that if you are beginning to see signs of memory loss, that your loved may also be aware of these same things. But denial may play a role in their perception as well as it does in yours. Instead of being realistically concerned about the potential problem the person may become irritable or depressed instead, or hypersensitive if their memory capacity is questioned in any way.

Then you have to learn one of the cardinal lessons of caregiving: **You have to be sooooo gentle!** Or put another way: Don't pounce!

Eventually however, you may wish to sit down with your loved one when both of you are relaxed and unhurried, and ask them if they have been aware of what you have noticed, and if they are concerned. If the answer is yes, you are well on your way to coming to grips with the problem, and the next step would be to schedule an initial medical evaluation with your loved one's primary care doctor. If the answer is no, it will be more difficult for you to deal with this emerging problem. He or she may become quite defensive, or irritated, or even accusatory, telling you that you are meddling in what is none of your business. Then it would be best to try to recruit allies, one or more other persons who have both you and your loved one's interest at heart, and to bring the matter up again, ever so gently. If none of this works you should discuss your concerns with your loved one's doctor at the next appointment. This process of coming to grips with the problem can take weeks or even months, sometimes years, before the problem is first confronted and then evaluated. Hopefully your persistent concern will be appreciated and acted upon. Again, as far as establishing a definitive diagnosis, this will be discussed in Chapter 7.

Get ready to take on the caregiver role.

Once you know that you are most likely dealing with Alzheimer's disease, it is time to get ready to take on the caregiver role. Keep in mind that when you become a caregiver it will be in addition to whatever else is going on in your life, whatever other roles you are playing, and whatever other obligations you already have. If this sounds heavy to you, it is. But doing anything new is difficult unless you learn all there is to know about the job. This includes two main goals: 1. Learning everything that you can about the disease you are dealing with in your loved one; and 2. Learning everything that you can about you, yourself, in the caregiver role. I am offering to be your coach on both of these topics.

So, in the next several chapters I am going to try to teach you everything you need to know about the disease. After that, I am going to try to teach you everything you need to know about yourself in the caregiver role.

Patients with Alzheimer's can also have other diseases.

Oh, one more thing. Patients with Alzheimer's can also have other diseases, such as diabetes, hypertension, arthritis, congestive heart failure, and so on. What that means is that in addition to being an Alzheimer's caregiver you may also have to take on helping your Alzheimer's patient manage their other diseases. I know you hadn't bargained for this. But unfortunately it, too, comes with the territory. This is particularly true as Alzheimer's disease progresses, as more and more of the tasks of managing the patient's other illness become yours to manage. Poorly controlled diabetes, hypertension, or heart disease, all will make the symptoms of Alzheimer's disease worse. So you are going to have to *become the patient's general health care manager as well.* As you read this, I can already hear you saying, "Thanks a bunch!"

Chapter Summary

1. **Alzheimer's disease affects memory and intellectual functioning**
2. **Behavioral problems can also occur.**

3. Know "The Seven Warning Signs of Alzheimer's Disease."

4. Become familiar with "The Short Portable Mental Status Questionnaire."

5. You are beginning to suspect it might be Alzheimer's disease.

6. Getting ready to take on the caregiver role.

7. Patients with Alzheimer's can also have other diseases.

8. So you are going to have to become their general healthcare manager as well.

Chapter Seven

Alzheimer's Disease Can Now Be Diagnosed

It is now possible to make a definite diagnosis of Alzheimer's disease

It used to be said that the diagnosis of Alzheimer's disease could only be made by performing a brain autopsy. While this was a perfectly reliable way of making the diagnosis, doing so after the patient had already died did not benefit either the patient or the caregiver. Today, however, it is possible to make the diagnosis of Alzheimer's disease in the living patient with a 90-95% accuracy. Moreover, the diagnosis can be made at every stage of the disease -- mild, moderate, or severe. It can even be made when the patient only has mild cognitive impairment, which we now regard as either a forerunner of Alzheimer's disease, or as the earliest stage of the disease.

What is needed to make a diagnosis of Alzheimer's?

Only a doctor, preferably one who is a specialist in memory disorders can make a definite diagnosis of Alzheimer's disease. In order to do so the doctor will need all of the following items:

- a detailed history of how memory problems have developed, obtained from both the patient and the caregiver
- a thorough general medical history

- a complete physical and neurological examination

- a battery of lab tests to include a complete blood count, tests of liver and kidney function, cholesterol and other lipid tests, and a fasting blood sugar

- a standard cardiogram (EKG)

- at least one imaging study of the brain, preferably an MRI scan of the brain, or a CAT scan, or even better, a PET scan of the brain

- an assessment of the degree of memory deficit, using one of the memory screening instruments such as the Mini-Mental Stratus Examination (Folstein MMSE) or the Short Portable Mental Status Questionnaire (Pfeiffer SPMSQ)

- in selective cases, a full-scale neuropsychological evaluation by a psychologist

- still more selectively, certain genetic tests, and measurement of A beta 42 amyloid and tau protein, in cerebrospinal fluid, blood or urine

Several of these tests require some additional explanation:

- When an MRI or CAT scan imaging study of the brain is performed, special emphasis needs to be placed on the appearance of the temporal lobe, particularly an area called the hippocampus and the amygdalar area. Atrophy in these areas is nearly completely specific to Alzheimer's disease

- When a PET scan of the brain is performed, additional information about the state of the brain will be obtained. A regular PET scan measures the amount of blood flow and glucose metabolism in the brain, with special emphasis on the temporal lobe where memory function occurs. Decreased blood flow and/or glucose metabolism is an early indicator of Alzheimer's disease. A still newer, modified PET scan is now beginning to come into use: *amyloid PET scanning*. Amyloid plaques in the brain are the most reliable hallmarks of Alzheimer's disease. Amyloid PET scanning measures the amount of amyloid plaques in the brain; the number of amyloid plaques seen, especially in the temporal and the frontal lobes of the brain, are a measure of the likelihood and the severity of the disease. While this type of scan is currently used for research purposes, it is likely that in the near future it will become a more regular part of a diagnostic workup for Alzheimer's disease.

- Neuropsychological testing should be performed when the results of other tests are inconclusive, or the person is only very mildly impaired, or is someone with a high level of education.

- Specific lab tests are further discussed below.

Laboratory test for Alzheimer's disease.

While it would be highly desirable to have a definitive lab test for Alzheimer's disease, none exists as yet. There are several lab tests that can contribute valuable information to the diagnostic process, however. But in the end, the diagnosis of Alzheimer's disease is still a clinical process, even though in experienced hands it can be 90-95% accurate, when compared with brain autopsy findings.

There are two major forms of Alzheimer's disease: 1. *Inherited Alzheimer's* disease which accounts for less than one half of one percent of all cases. This form of the disease generally starts in individuals in their forties, and patients with this form of the disease generally die in their fifties or early sixties. Exactly fifty percent of the off-spring of these individuals will also develop the disease, and genetic DNA testing can reveal whether a child of such an individual has that gene. This is a complex ethical question. Should such individual be tested at an early age and thereby find out whether they will or will not develop the disease? Genetic counseling is definitely indicated in these situations. 2. *Spontaneous Alzheimer's* disease accounts for almost all other cases of Alzheimer's disease. The disease begins only rarely when someone is in their sixties, and more commonly starts when people are in their seventies, eighties, and nineties. Age is the greatest risk factor for spontaneous Alzheimer's disease, i.e. the risk increases with advancing age, and family history plays only a relatively minor role. But in these cases a genetic test, the ApoE test may have a possible role to play.

You may not need to know all the details about this test, but if you or your doctor are considering using this test, it may be good to have this information (if the ApoE test is not at all being considered for your loved one, you may skip the rest of this paragraph). The ApoE test determines whether an individual has one or more of the genes that favor development of Alzheimer's disease. There are three variants of the ApoE gene: ApoE 2 is protective against Alzheimer's disease; ApoE 3 is relatively neutral; ApoE 4 favors the development of Alzheimer's. Each individual inherits one ApoE gene from their mother, and one from their father. Carriers of one ApoE 4 gene have a slightly higher risk for developing the disease than do persons without any ApoE 4 gene. Carriers of two ApoE 4 genes have a significantly greater risk of developing the disease, estimated at almost 70 percent. Today the ApoE test is used primarily as a research tool, not as a clinically useful diagnostic tool. The reason for this is that people without any ApoE 4 gene can still develop Alzheimer's. More than half of those with two ApoE genes will develop the disease eventually. But the ApoE gene is only a *risk factor* for developing the disease and not a determining factor. As I have said, the biggest risk factor for developing the spontaneous form of Alzheimer's disease is advancing age, not heredity.

Other types of lab tests exist which have some usefulness in the diagnostic process. These measure the level of various chemical compounds relevant to Alzheimer's disease, either in the urine, the blood, or in cerebrospinal fluid. *Amyloid plaques,* made up of clumps of A-beta amyloid protein, and *fibrillary tangles*, made up of tau proteins, are the most specific findings of Alzheimer's disease in the brain. Tests for levels of these compounds currently form the basis for spinal fluid, blood, and urine tests for Alzheimer's disease. Currently, the most sensitive test for Alzheimer's is a spinal fluid test for these chemicals: an elevated level of tau protein and a decreased level of A-beta 42 protein are found in patients with established Alzheimer's disease. Such a finding can *support* a clinical diagnosis of Alzheimer's disease, but by itself is not diagnostic. Tests which measure similar compounds in the blood and urine are also sometimes used to *support* a clinical diagnosis, but by themselves are not definitive.

The majority of experts on Alzheimer's disease feel that such lab tests are at this time used primarily as *research tools*, and they are not recommended for routine use in making a diagnosis of Alzheimer's disease.

Elements of the diagnosis you as the caregiver need to know

When your loved one has had a complete diagnostic evaluation what are the elements of the diagnosis that you as a caregiver need to know? Here are the questions to which you should receive relatively clear answers:

1. Are you definitely dealing with Alzheimer's disease, yes or no?

2. Or are you dealing with Alzheimer's disease **plus** something else, such as a mixture of Alzheimer's and vascular dementia?

3. Or are you dealing with something other than Alzheimer's disease, such as vascular dementia, or Lewy-Body dementia, or post traumatic or post encephalitic dementia?

4. Assuming that you are definitely dealing with Alzheimer's disease, what will be the rate of progression, slow, intermediate, or rapid?

5. In addition to memory and intellectual impairment, are you also dealing with behavioral problems? These can be more troublesome than memory problems, and may require separate interventions.

You will need to know the answer to all of these questions so that you can make appropriate plans, both for your loved one and for yourself.

Chapter Summary

1. **Only a doctor, preferably a specialist in memory disorders, can make a definite diagnosis of Alzheimer's disease.**

2. **Know what is needed to make a definitive diagnosis of Alzheimer's disease.**

3. **Know the value and the limitations of laboratory test for diagnosing Alzheimer's disease.**

Chapter Eight

Alzheimer's Disease Can Now Be Treated

Alzheimer's disease can now be treated

Until the *1990s* there was no treatment for Alzheimer's. However, real progress has been made in this area as a result of research. Therefore treatment should now be started as soon as the diagnosis has been definitively established. The reason for this is that the effect of treatment is basically to reduce present symptoms and *to slow the progression of the disease*. Thus, starting treatment as soon as possible will have the best chance to preserve the highest level of function in the affected individual. Any delay in starting treatment will produce less favorable results since the disease will have progressed further and the starting level of the patient's function will then be much lower.

The currently available treatments do not cure the disease, but this is true of the vast majority of chronic diseases. Thus, for instance, even after successful treatment to control diabetes, the patient will still have diabetes. After successful treatment of Alzheimer's disease, the patient will still have Alzheimer's disease, but the symptoms will be less severe and the rate of progression will have slowed significantly. It is also extremely important that the diagnosis be made as early as possible, as that will have the greatest chance of retaining near normal functioning in the affected individual. At the same time, it will also ease the burden of care on the caregiver.

Medications for Treating Alzheimer's Disease

There are now two classes of medication available for the treatment of Alzheimer's disease. They are categorized as *cholinesterase inhibitors* and *NMDA-inhibitors* respectively. Included in the first class are the drugs *Aricept, Exelon, and Razadyne,* and in the second class there is only one drug available, called *Namenda.* The two classes of drugs work by entirely different mechanisms, which means that when they are used together they can produce a greater benefit than when either category of drug is given alone. In fact, the combination of Aricept and Namenda was shown in one study to produce greater benefit in terms of memory function, self-care capacity and disruptive behaviors than could be obtained with Aricept alone. The FDA has approved the use of Aricept, Exelon, and Razadyne for mild and moderate Alzheimer's disease, while Namenda has been approved for moderate and severe Alzheimer's disease. Aricept has also been approved for continued use into severe stages of Alzheimer's disease. For descriptions of what constitutes mild, moderate, and severe Alzheimer's disease, please familiarize yourself with all the information contained in Chapters 9 through 11. Treatment should be begun as soon as the diagnosis has been made, starting with one of the cholinesterase inhibitors in the mild stages, and adding Namenda in the middle (moderate) and late (severe) stages. Treatment with these medications should then continue until late into the disease.

These medications are not a cure for the disease, but they can first *improve* and later on *slow the progression* of memory problems, of self-care capacity, and of disruptive behaviors. Combination therapy with these medications can also help to maintain communication skills on the part of the patient.

Intense research efforts are currently under way to test several new medications, with yet differing mechanisms of action. These newer medications may be able to bring about additional benefits and further slow the progression of the disease. Accordingly, it will be important for you to watch for announcements of such additional breakthroughs.

Participation in Clinical Studies

In the meantime, before additional medications to treat Alzheimer's become available to the general public, you can try to enroll your loved one in one or more clinical studies. Clinical studies are being conducted in multiple research centers across the US, and one or another of these may be taking place in your community. You can locate such studies by going on the internet, and using such search engines as Google.com or Bing.com, and entering the phrase "Alzheimer's disease, clinical studies." Your doctor may also be aware of where these studies are conducted, or you can contact a chapter of the Alzheimer's Association in your community.

There are a number of distinct advantages to having your loved participate in a clinical study. These include:

- access to new medications before they become available to the general public

- state of the art diagnostic evaluations

- access to a complete research team deeply knowledgeable about the disease

- extensive ongoing care for patients and caregivers

Participation in most clinical studies is at no cost to the patient or caregiver. Some studies even provide reimbursement for the cost of travel to the site.

There can also be some disadvantages to participation in clinical studies:

- Not everyone wishing to participate may be eligible, as criteria for participation vary. Individuals with certain illnesses or those taking specific medications may be excluded.

- Clinical studies are generally "randomized, double-blind, placebo controlled" studies. What this means is that your loved one may be on a placebo (inactive) medication for a portion of time in the study. Neither you nor your loved one will know whether or not they are actually getting the active medication until the end of the study.

- Since medications in these studies have not yet been approved for this use, there is the possibility of adverse side effects. However, be assured that patients in such studies are very closely monitored for the occurrence of any side effects.

On the whole, advantages of participating in clinical studies far outweigh any of the disadvantages. And you and your loved one may have the distinction of making a real contribution to discovering a new treatment for Alzheimer's disease.

Medications to treat behavioral problems

The medications we have discussed so far can help reduce some behavioral problems, such as depression, irritability, or agitation. But if these problems are more severe, additional medications are available to treat them. They include antidepressant medications for severe depression, and major tranquilizers for severe agitation or for hallucinations and delusions. If these should be needed, your treating doctor can further explain and if needed prescribe them for your loved one. Only some patients with this disease will show behavioral problems, so this may or may not be relevant to your situation.

Non-medicinal treatments in Alzheimer's disease

There are also a number of non-medicinal treatments available for Alzheimer's disease. These can include memory-training classes, especially in the early stages of the disease. Vigorous physical exercise has also been proven to be remarkably beneficial in improving memory as well as behavioral problems.

The most critical element of any treatment program: You, the caregiver

Finally, we come to discuss what is clearly the most critical component of any treatment program for someone with Alzheimer's disease: you, the caregiver. An informed, trained, and committed caregiver is what is needed most. The remainder of this book is devoted to helping you become that caregiver.

And to the extent that I do not cover everything that you will need to know or do, I will refer you to additional resource persons or agencies in your own community.

For how long will you need to be a caregiver?

Alzheimer's disease is an extremely variable disease. It can last anywhere from two to twenty-five years. So for how long are you going to have to be a caregiver? While no one can give you a precise answer to that question, it is possible to give you a very good estimate concerning the patient you are caring for specifically. This is not done by magic but by good and careful observation on the part of you and your loved one's doctor. For instance, if the patient has only reached the mild or early stages of the disease, then one can judge that the patient is pursuing a slow course, and that the entire illness may last anywhere from 15 to 20 years. If on the other hand the patient has already reached the severe stages in two to three years from start of the first symptoms, then he or she may be expected to run the entire course of the illness in as little as four to five years. Most commonly, however, the entire course of the disease can take from seven to ten years, from first symptoms to final outcome. So, with that knowledge you can more adequately prepare yourself mentally and practically for the length of time that you are going to be in the caregiver role.

Chapter Summary

1. **Understand that Alzheimer's is now a treatable disease.**

2. **Become familiar with current medications for Alzheimer's.**

3. **Consider participating in clinical studies in Alzheimer's disease.**

4. **Understand medications for the treatment of behavioral problems.**

5. **Be aware of non-medicinal treatments in Alzheimer's.**

6. **Finally, recognize the most important element in any treatment plan for Alzheimer's: It is you, the caregiver.**

7. The remainder of this book is devoted to letting you become the consummate caregiver for your loved one.

8. Understand for how long you may need to be a caregiver.

Chapter Nine

Caregiving in the Early Stages of Alzheimer's

Early on in the disease, you are a "caregiver-in-waiting"

In the earliest stages of Alzheimer's, when both you and your loved one are still just trying to figure out what is happening, we cannot even speak of you as "the caregiver." Assuming the role of caregiver requires a delicate negotiation to establish that someone is in need of care, and that isn't at all clear early on. As I have said before, "you have to be soooo gentle." Many an individual in the early stages of the disease has blurted out, sometimes with some degree of anger, "I don't need a caregiver." And for the most part they are right. At this stage the affected individual can still pretty much do everything they need or want to do: drive a car, make a telephone call, socialize, cook a meal, dress and groom themselves. In fact, you are only a "caregiver in waiting," waiting to step in *if* you are needed, and not otherwise. You haven't been "commissioned" yet.

As it becomes clearer to both of you where help is needed, you can offer that help and then again step back, when it is clear that nothing further is required. This kind of back-and-forth is likely to go on for weeks and months, as the diagnosis is pursued, established, and possible treatment is initiated.

Work with an elder law attorney

During this time, before problems become more serious, you also need to plan while you and your loved one can plan jointly, to prepare for the weeks, months, and years ahead. I recommend that you do this with the help of an elder law attorney who is familiar with all the important documents that need to be drawn up before your loved one becomes so disabled that he or she can no longer participate in this process.

Obtain a durable family power of attorney.

One of the first tasks to be accomplished is to have your loved one give you power-of-attorney. This will allow your loved one to make decisions for themselves for as long as they are able; that authority will then pass on to you when they are no longer able to do so. You will also want to establish yourself or another trusted member of the family to be appointed as healthcare surrogate, to make needed medical decisions related to Alzheimer's or other illnesses throughout the remainder of your loved one's life. This is also an excellent time and probably the last time, to review your loved one's will, and to amend it, if necessary. Please review also the section of power of attorney and on testamentary capacity in the Appendix of this book. Do not be surprised if bringing up these subjects stirs up some initial resistance or anxiety, not only in your loved one, but in you, the caregiver, as well. But these are absolutely vital steps you will need to take together with your loved one. And once again, you have to be soooo gentle and so patient!

During the early stages of this disease it should be your goal to keep life flowing in as normal a way as possible, although both you and your loved one know that change has come and more change is coming. Exactly what that means will, of course, depend on how you have been living your lives together up to this time. It may evoke in you or your loved one a desire to take an inventory of what all you still want to do while it is still possible: take a cruise, see Europe, and spend time with the grandchildren, what have you. You can create your own "bucket list." (If you are not familiar with this term, it means deciding what you still want to do, separately or together before either one of you "kicks the bucket.)" In the case of Alzheimer's disease it is not so much a matter of before either one of you dies, but before one of you becomes so disabled that certain activities might no longer be possible. Again, this is a very delicate exploration. The mutual love and trust that has been built between you and your loved one will make this as easy as is possible under the circumstances.

If your loved one, however, is unwilling or unable to admit that change is coming, i.e. if he or she is in denial, the job becomes a lot harder. I have seen quite a few people, particularly people who have been powerful and prominent in their community, reject any admission that something is wrong, and then of course both of you are in real trouble. Your loved one won't avail himself or herself of the treatment that is needed, and preparation for the future will not take place. Consult with the doctor about how this might best be overcome, or, if you are already attending a caregiver support group, (which we will discuss shortly) ask your peers in the group how they may have overcome a similar problem.

Should your loved one be told that they have Alzheimer's disease?

This is indeed a very important question, but one for which there is no easy answer. You as the caregiver should certainly know that you are dealing with Alzheimer's. But as it relates to the affected individual, the answer is not so clear. In my medical practice, I have not had a hard and fast rule about this, but rather have been guided by the circumstances of the particular case. If someone asked me whether they have Alzheimer's disease, I have generally asked what they know about the disease and whether they think they have the disease. Some individuals would be extremely threatened by hearing this diagnosis applied to them, and in those cases I have generally told them that they "have a memory problem," that I am extremely interested in helping them with that problem, that we now have medication to treat memory problems, and they then may have to rely on other people, their spouse, their children etc., to help them with certain decisions and activities. If someone appears to be capable of accepting the Alzheimer's disease diagnosis, I will say that they "probably" have Alzheimer's disease, leaving a ray of hope that it just might be something else. The reason for handling this issue with a certain degree of discretion is that some individuals have a really negative, scary view of what Alzheimer's disease is. Occasionally someone has even attempted suicide when they were told of the diagnosis, without having been given the information about treatments available, and how to live with Alzheimer's. But one way or another the affected person must be told that they have a serious memory problem, and what the implications of that might be, including the availability of treatment and support. So from here on forward you will know whether your loved one understands that they are either dealing with "a memory problem" or that they "probably" have Alzheimer's disease.

Now you are ready to become an official caregiver.

So now that you have been told that your loved one has Alzheimer's disease, and your loved one has more or less accepted that they either have a serious "memory problem" or that they "probably" have Alzheimer's disease, now you are ready to step into the caregiver role officially. During these early stages of the disease, the demands made on the caregiver are relatively modest. Patients are still able to communicate effectively with the caregiver; they are able to perform all the basic as well as the more complex activities of daily living (eating, dressing, grooming, making purchases, using transportation, including driving their own automobile, using the telephone and so on. However, when it comes to short-term memory their performance falls short. They may forget appointments, they may not be able to deliver a message they took over the phone, and they may forget to take their prescribed medication. So what is needed on the part of the caregiver is a kind of a hovering presence that allows the patient to do what they can still do, but is ready to step in and provide assistance when it is needed. Put another way, the number of hours you will actually be doing specific things for your loved will be relatively few. However, your role as a hovering "guardian angel" will be in operation 24/7. Yes, caregiving really is the original or the quintessential 24/7, or 24/7/365 job. Take a deep breath.

Caregiving is a job: it requires a plan and a schedule

It may be useful to think of caregiving as a kind of job. You have to take it seriously, you have to plan, and you have to have a schedule. It is not like any other job, but I've already told you that. Remember 24/7/365? So what do you do first, and what do you do next, and what do you do after that? Good questions. Not so easy to answer.

To start with, you need to be a keen observer. Look for what is changed, and then decide if there is something you need to do about it. Not all changes you may see will require a specific response. Let me try to help organize your observations: Changes are likely to happen in four areas: 1. memory; 2. communications; 3. routine everyday activities; and 4. troublesome changes in mood or behavior.

1. Changes in memory: During this phase of the disease you are likely to discover that memory for recent events, recent conversations, and updating of events or times, will be the most prominent changes. You may find yourself having to repeat conversations you have had, or you may need to answer the same question more than once. Keeping track of the day of the week and the date, since these require constant updating, may slip fairly easily. You may want to keep the day of the week and the date displayed somewhere prominently in your home to help with orientation. If your loved one does make mistakes, it is important that you respond to them *with equanimity,* rather than with annoyance.

2. Changes in communications: You may observe that your loved one will not finish a sentence, or may get stuck on trying to find a word that simply won't come out. If you understand enough of the sentence, you don't need to do anything. If you can guess what word your loved one is trying to say, go ahead and supply the word, so that the conversation can continue. For example: if your loved is saying: "We have to go to the ....(can't come up with the name)," go ahead and say "the Williams's" so that your loved one can complete the sentence. This will be less frustrating than if you are waiting for the right name to emerge.

3. Everyday activities: Let us say your spouse starts to mow the lawn or to wash the dishes, but doesn't finish the job. There is no need to make a big deal

out of it. Ask your spouse to please start again on the same task (remember: you have to be soooo gentle!) or finish the job yourself. We'll come to concerns about driving a little later on.

4. Changes in mood or behavior: if you notice your loved one becoming blue or irritable, try to initiate a new activity with him or her. Suggest something that you know they usually really like to do, like: "let's go for a walk, it is such a beautiful day today," or "let's have a picnic out in the back yard today." Or offer a compliment that you can sincerely make, such as "you're wearing such a nice outfit today," or "I sure appreciate your helping me put away the dishes today."

Next, you need to make a plan or a schedule for each day

It turns out that having a similar routine of activities each day works best for persons in the early, and even in the later stages of this disease. What that routine will consist of depends on what routines the person has followed before they developed the disease. You might think that routines would become boring, but they can actually be quite comfortable. Routines around meal times are probably the simplest and most reliable schedule to establish. After that, try to ask your loved one to do a task that he or she can still easily perform, and then thank them for doing that task. Simple? Right.

Schedule at least one really pleasurable activity every day

This is an important suggestion. Try to find an activity that both you and your loved can enjoy. It could be a walk in the park, playing a game of cards, cooking a meal together, exercising together, playing with your dog or cat, going shopping for groceries, dancing, listening to music, watching a favorite video, or any number of other things. In our city, one of the theme parks allows people to purchase an admission ticket one time and to return as often as they wish throughout the year. So, for instance a visit to Busch Gardens, or SeaWorld, or the aquarium, or your local park or museum, might be something you could do repeatedly. Another thing that many patients with Alzheimer's disease enjoy is looking through photo albums of relatives and friends, or photos of an earlier period in your lives. If you yourself can't think of any such activities, talk to other caregivers about what is working for them and their loved ones. Which brings me to one of the most important bits of advice that I can give you:

At the earliest possible time, join a caregiver support group

You will find that joining an Alzheimer's caregiver support group will be a real life-saver for you. You will first of all see that you are not alone in struggling with some of these problems. Second, you will have an opportunity to learn from other caregivers what they have found that worked with their loved ones. You will also enjoy the camaraderie of being with people who are in the same boat as you are. How do you find a caregiver group? The doctor or clinic to whom you are taking your loved one is likely to know of such a group. If not, you can call your local Area Agency on Aging, or your local chapter of the Alzheimer's Association, or your local hospital, to find out when and where such groups are conducted. A caregiver group usually consists of a group facilitator who may be a memory specialist, a social worker, nurse, or doctor, or even a lay leader, plus a dozen or more people who are dealing with various stages of caregiving for their loved one. Generally there is absolutely no cost to attend. Sometimes a support group even has an activity program in which your loved one can participate while you attend the group session. Or you can learn about caregiver groups by going on the internet, typing in "Alzheimer's support group", followed by the name of your community, and you're likely to find a listing there. Later on, when you yourself have become an experienced caregiver, and have discovered some things that work really well with your patient, you will be able to pass on these "secrets" to other caregivers in the group. You will find that they will be very grateful to you for your advice.

Dealing with mood and behavioral problems

Behavioral problems are generally quite mild at this stage of the disease. They tend to stem from the fact that your loved one is quite aware that they are not functioning as well as they once did, and these may be their reactions. There may be some mild depression or irritability, or a lack of interest in initiating or completing activities. A generally loving and supportive attitude towards the patient will alleviate many of these relatively minor problems. If more serious mood or behavior problems crop up, discuss them with the doctor or bring them up for discussion in your support group.

Dealing with changes in hygiene and toileting

At this stage of the disease, problems in this area tend to be relatively mild also. Here the word "prompting" will become very important to you. You may need to prompt your loved to change clothes, to take a bath, and so on. At this stage the person generally still has full control of bodily functions such as getting to the bathroom on time. But this will become an area of much greater concern in the middle and late stages of the disease.

Dealing with secondary caregivers and other interested parties

Not that you don't have enough to deal with already, there is one other area to which I need to call your attention, i.e., secondary caregivers. What I mean by that is that other members of your family have an interest in the well-being of your loved one: your children, a brother or sister, an in-law or other "interested parties." These individuals may at times tell you that you should be doing something else for your loved one than what you are doing. Your role as the primary caregiver of your loved one will always be to listen, and to consider whatever advice is given but *you* need to be the one to decide whether to heed that advice or not. One of the ways of dealing with such advice is to ask the person giving you advice to participate in the caregiving process, perhaps to spell you for an afternoon so that you can attend to some other things. This can at times get quite emotional. Let us say your daughter thinks that you should admit your spouse to a nursing home, or some other suggestion, and you clearly disagree. There are no simple answers to this situation. Discuss the issue with the doctor or with members of your caregiver group, and if there is disagreement, bring the opinion of these other "experts" to bear on the issue. As I have said, listen always. Consider, always, but comply only when the advice really makes sense to you and/or to the doctor or your group of peers in your support group.

Above all, continue to take great care of yourself

Above all, you need to continue to take great care of yourself, both for your own sake as well as for the sake of your loved one. You cannot afford to neglect your own health care, beauty care, leisure activities, rest and recreation, and so on. If you go "down the tubes" your loved one is sure to follow. So you need to make time for yourself, in this stage of the disease, and even more importantly later. So it may be well for you to take an advance look at the chapters on"Caregivers Need Care, Too," and begin to follow the advice contained therein. Both you and your loved one will benefit.

Chapter Summary

1. Early on in the process, you are still only a "caregiver-in-waiting."

2. Decide whether your loved needs to be told that they have Alzheimer's disease.

3. Now you are ready to become an official caregiver.

4. Caregiving is a job: it requires a plan and a schedule.

5. Make a plan and a schedule for each day.

6. Schedule at least one pleasurable activity each day.

7. At the earliest possible time, join a support group.

8. Learn how to deal with memory problems.

9. Learn how to deal with mood and behavioral problems.

10. Learn how to deal with changes in hygiene.

11. Learn how to deal with secondary caregivers and other interested parties.

12. Above all, continue to take great care of yourself.

Chapter Ten

Caregiving in the Middle Stages of Alzheimer's

Caregiving becomes tougher as the disease progresses

Yes, caregiving becomes tougher as the disease progresses. Many more areas of the patient's functioning are now affected. Patients may now experience not only short-term but long-term memory loss as well. Just in case it is not clear what is meant by long-term memory, let me give you a couple of illustrations. The person with long-term memory problems, when asked what their job had been, might reply that they had a very good job, or that they worked very hard, rather than being able to name their specific position or occupation. When asked where they went to college, they might reply that they went to college "up North," or that they went to a very good college. Patients in the middle stages of Alzheimer's disease will now require more assistance with everyday activities: they may not be able to use the TV remote, or set the thermostat properly, or use a microwave oven, or perform other complex tasks. They certainly should no longer be operating a motor vehicle. Please see the section on driving in the Appendix. Behavior problems may also become more severe, requiring increasingly more creative responses on the part of the caregiver. Irritability and hostility may crop up with greater frequency. There may be lapses of tact, such as calling a fat person fat to their face, or making inappropriate sexual overtures to acquaintances. Even though symptoms and deficits may be much more apparent now, a certain degree of denial will continue. Patients will tend to minimize or downplay their problems. Occasionally however, the gravity of the problem may sink in and patients may become seriously depressed.

Some of the same caregiver strategies used in the mild stages of the disease still apply, perhaps in somewhat altered form. 1. You still have to be *soooo* gentle! 2. The need for structure and routine continues or has, if anything, increased. 3. You still need to engage the patient in at least one pleasurable activity every day, although the nature of that activity may have to change. Overall, caregivers can expect to spend many more hours each day and each week, doing something for or with the patient. Increasingly, there is a need for the caregiver to share the burden of care with someone else, or to "outsource" some of the caregiving. Let us now discuss some specific elements of worsening symptoms and greater need for caregiver involvement:

How to cope with worsening memory problems

As both short-term (recent) and long-term (remote) memory become increasingly impaired, the caregiver will need to serve as surrogate memory to the patient, filling in blank spaces where needed, or glossing over the issue of failed memory. Nothing is to be gained by dwelling on the fact that the patient cannot remember the information. Nor is there any benefit in correcting the patient when they mis-remember something that the caregiver knows is not true. When meeting people, the caregiver should clearly identify the person they are meeting, rather than assuming that the patient remembers with whom he is speaking.

Also, please note that from here on, in this chapter and also in the next chapter, I will be referring to the person affected by Alzheimer's disease as "the patient." I also recommend that you begin to think of your loved one in more objective, clinical terms, and not just as "my spouse" or "my mother" or "my father." This may enable you to respond to any troublesome behaviors more objectively rather than just emotionally.

How to cope with worsening hygiene and toileting problems

In the area of personal hygiene, you as the caregiver may now need to prompt and supervise much more closely the patient's grooming and dressing. Always give the patient only single, simple instructions, instead of stringing a whole series of instructions together. For instance, you can say: "now put the tooth paste on your toothbrush." Wait for that action to be accomplished before going on to the next instruction. Still later on you may need to perform these activities *for* the patient altogether. In terms of their getting to the bathroom on time, it will be best to establish a routine of taking the patient to the toilet roughly every two hours, "whether they need it or not," in order to avoid embarrassing urinary incontinence. Some patients even begin to urinate in inappropriate places, such as in a waste basket, and even closer supervision is then indicated.

How to cope with worsening behavioral problems

During this phase of the disease behavioral problems tend to multiply. And if you are like most caregivers, you will find the behavioral problems far more challenging than "mere" memory problems. Some patients, but by no means all of them, may now experience episodes of anxiety, depression or agitation. Even worse, you may see irritability or outright hostility expressed towards the caregiver. If this should happen with your patient, you will need to acquire a number of new skills and techniques to diffuse, redirect, and stop the undesired activity. Examples of these might be the following: When a patient first begins to express hostility towards the caregiver or even threatens to hit the caregiver, immediate strong countermeasures need to be taken: First of all, protect yourself at all costs, and in any way you can. Being hurt or injured by the person you are caring for is not part of your agreement to be a caregiver.

Amazingly, barking back at the patient in the manner of a drill sergeant often aborts the angry attack. Or you may even need to call for help from a neighbor or even the police; or you can threaten to stop being the person's caregiver. One caregiver said to her angry husband: "If you ever do this again, I am going to send you to a nursing home." The patient stopped attacking her, and she never had to say it again.

Other techniques may include distracting or redirecting the patient. R*edirecting is more effective than distracting.* Redirecting means inviting the patient to enter upon an entirely different activity: "Let's go for a walk. Let's go to McDonald's or some other suggestion that might be appealing to the patient.

Also, during this stage hallucinations *and*/or delusions may make their appearance for the first time. Hallucinations and/or delusions may be of two types that have very different meanings and require a different type of response. The first type of hallucinations or delusions consists of images, voices, or beliefs that are what I call *innocent* distortions of reality. They tend to "re-animate" the world of the patient with interesting but harmless visions, voices, or beliefs. One example of this might be a patient who complained that a cow was regularly coming into the living room. The patient sees the cow but you do not. The patient however is not afraid of the cow and is not threatened by the fact that there is a cow in his living room. A *dangerous hallucination or delusion* is one in which the patient feels threatened by the imagined vision, voice, or belief, and is intent on defending himself against it. This requires a very different kind of response. For the latter you need to consult with the patient's doctor who may be able to prescribe a major tranquilizer or even give an injection. For the innocent hallucination you have two choices: you can either go along with the hallucination without contradicting the patient, or you can become creative as the caregiver did whose husband saw the cow in his living room. She agreed with him that there was a cow, and said to her husband, "Let's open the door and push the cow out of the room." She opened the door, pushed the cow out of the living room, and her husband was satisfied. The vision of the cow never returned.

Using a sense of humor

Being able to respond to things with a sense of humor is a wonderful technique for anyone under any circumstances, but it is particularly useful to caregivers looking after an Alzheimer's patient. That does not mean that you are laughing at the patient or their behavior, but that you can and do see the funny aspects of any occurrence. One caregiver wrote down the following story for me about an event with her mother:

An Afternoon at the Beach

Well, I guess by now you know my mom has Alzheimer's disease. Until about six months ago she was living with John, but that ended when he couldn't deal with her wetting and soiling herself. So she came to live with me.

I try to do things with Mom. We have a place by the beach, and I asked if she wanted to go.

"Great," she said, "let's go."

We had a nice drive to the beach. We went up to our condominium, and I asked her if she wanted to go for a walk on the beach.

"Yep," she said, "let's go"

I unpacked my swim suit and hers. We both have one-piece bathing suits, both of them blue with some other colors mixed in. I went into the bathroom to change and handed her her bathing suit to put on.

When I came out I saw that something looked funny. She turned around and I realized that she had put her bathing suit on front to back!

"Mom." I started to yell at her, "you've got your bathing suit on backwards!" But I quickly realized that yelling at her was not going to helpful. So I changed course. I took her over to the mirror, but she still didn't quite understand. She tried to hide her breasts behind the slim back straps, but it didn't quite work. So I helped her put on her bathing suit the right way. We both had a good laugh then and went out for a nice walk on the beach, as though nothing had happened. Well, I guess nothing had happened."

By making a light-hearted moment out of the occasion, the caregiver easily diffused the situation instead of treating it as a disaster.

Coping with loss of social inhibitions

When social disinhibitions crop up you need to be somewhat prepared for the effect this may have on other people, whether this be the making of inappropriate remarks, or less than optimal eating behavior (like eating food with one's fingers, for example). You may want to have cards printed up that you can give to onlookers, restaurant serving personnel, or even strangers, saying something like this: "Please excuse my loved one's behavior. He suffers from a memory disorder (Alzheimer's disease)." These cards can then be subtly slipped to the stranger, etc. so that they understand what is happening.

Failure to recognize the caregiver

One of the most poignant events that can occur in the middle stages of Alzheimer's disease is the moment that the patient fails to recognize the caregiver. He or she may be perceived as a total stranger, or as another member of the patient's family, a son or a daughter or parent or some other person close to the patient. Many caregivers are devastated when this happens. After all that they are doing and have done for the patient, the patient no longer recognizes the caregiver! Well, be prepared; it may happen to you at some time during the caregiving process, or it may not, but if it happens to another caregiver, perhaps you can comfort them and explain to them that the patient is simply mistaking the caregiver for someone else dear to them. Or that he remembers her as that beautiful young woman she was when you first met, and she probably doesn't look exactly like that anymore. The patient has gone back to some meaningful image in their past. You may need to be prepared for this. Have in mind reminding your patient of some particularly meaningful moment in your relationship that only *you* could know. Retell the event to the patient and tell them that you are the one that he or she surely remembers from that meaningful event. The patient may have an "ahah!" moment and recognize you again, or you may need to let time pass and wait for another time when he or she will recognize you for who you are. Do not be dismayed, this is not your failure; it is the disease speaking, not your loved one. That's why I wanted to alert you to this possibility so that you should not feel so hurt.

Oh, there are so many more problems that can crop up.

Yes, there are many more challenges that can develop in the months and years of your caregiving experience. I cannot predict all of them for you. Keep an open mind, and try to understand what might be happening in the mind of your loved one when something unforeseen happens. "Let not your heart be troubled, neither let it be afraid," as the Bible says. And if you develop some new technique for coping with unforeseen problems, share your wisdom with other caregivers. You can save them some trouble, and they will be grateful to you. Remember, I never promised you a rose garden.

Chapter Summary

1. **Caregiving becomes tougher as the disease progresses.**

2. **Learn how to cope with worsening memory problems.**

3. **Learn how to cope with worsening hygiene and toileting problems.**

4. **Learn how to cope with worsening behavioral problems.**

5. Hone your sense of humor; it is essential.

6. Learn to cope with social disinhibitions.

7. Prepare for the time when the patient fails to recognize you.

8. There are so many more challenges that can crop up.

9. And remember, I never promised you a rose garden

Chapter Eleven

Caregiving in the Late Stages of Alzheimer's

In the late stages of the disease more and more abilities disappear, and the behavioral problems become much worse. The task of being a caregiver becomes much more challenging, both in kind and in quantity. So here you will need all the help you can get.

Memory problems are now much worse

First of all, of course, memory problems have now become much worse, both for recent events and for long-ago happenings. Things you may have just said to your loved one will not be remembered, and you may have to repeat them time and again. Also, the meaning of words begins to disappear. Not only will your patient not be able to understand exactly what you have said, but they themselves will not be able to find words. They may know exactly what they want to say, but will not be able to produce the word they are looking for. They may point to a watch or a clock, but not be able to say the words "watch" or "clock."

As already discussed in the previous chapter, there will now be times when your loved one will no longer be able to recognize you. They may mistake your for someone else or for a stranger, and in fact become frightened of you if they misinterpret who you are. This is really tough when someone you have lived with and loved for fifty years no longer knows who you are.

Even more troublesome will be the fact that the person you are caring for may at times no longer even recognize *themselves*. They may see themselves in the mirror and ask: "What is that old man (or that old woman) doing in my bathroom?" Just to give you an idea of how to respond to this challenging situation, you may need to cover the mirrors in your bathroom with towels until this phase of the disease passes.

Verbal communications are now quite limited

Verbal communications in this phase of the disease will have become quite limited. "Yes" and "no" may be the only words the person can form regularly, and they may develop a kind of short-hand to express themselves. For instance, one patient used just the single word "McDonald's" to indicate that he wanted to be taken to McDonalds for a hamburger. You will have to learn to guess or interpret what the patient is trying to tell you. If the patient can't find a word when trying to tell you something, supply the missing word to the patient, if you can guess it, so the conversation can continue. Nothing is gained by insisting that the patient try to come up with the missing word. You would only have created additional frustration.

Behavioral problems become more prominent

And as in the middle stages of the disease, there may be hallucinations and delusions. Hallucinations occur when the patient sees or hears something or someone whom you yourself cannot see or hear. Most of the time, these sensations are relatively benign and do not disturb the patient, although they may be upsetting to you. At other times, the patient may become severely frightened in response to these hallucinations, feeling they are in danger or that they are being attacked. When this occurs, you will need to consult with the treating physician to see if additional medication, or a tranquilizer, may be indicated to help the patient get over this. More often, however, hallucinations are merely interesting to the patient rather than frightening. One of my patients used to see children coming into his living room, and his interpretation was that they were coming into this room because it was the only room in the house that was air-conditioned.

Still more troublesome can be delusions. One patient of mine regularly accused her caregiver husband of stealing her clothes from her closet. She would become very angry, go to complain about her husband to the neighbors, or sometimes even call the police. This caregiver husband was one of the most caring, loving, gentle persons you could imagine, but when his wife could not find something that she had misplaced, the accusations began. This situation required her doctor to prescribe increasing doses of a major tranquilizer. After several increases in the dose of the medication, the delusions disappeared, and she once again began to sing the praises of her husband whom she described as "the best caregiver ever."

Another change in behavior may occur at this stage of the disease. The patient may experience either depression or apathy. Spontaneous activities will grind to a halt; the patient will not eat, get dressed, or participate in any activities. Trying to distract the patient or offering tender loving care may help, but sometimes medications will be needed. Again bring this to the doctor's attention. So you can see, at this stage of the disease you may have to be in frequent contact with your patient's doctor, or consult with members of your support group who may have developed some skill or technique for dealing with one of the many behavioral problems which can occur.

Sleep disturbances, including a complete reversal of day-night cycle, is another troublesome behavior that may occur. And if your patient cannot sleep, you are not going to be able to sleep either, which will very quickly run you down physically and emotionally. You may need to get help from friends or relatives to care for the patient for some hours while you get some sleep. Exercise or other physical activity during day time hours may be helpful in providing more regular sleep for the patient, but again, temporary use of sleep-inducing medication may be needed. This is not without risk, as sleeping medications can further impair the patient's memory function and lead to unsteadiness of gait, day time drowsiness, and the risk of falls. Nothing could be worse for a patient with Alzheimer's disease than to experience a hip fracture or similar mishap. Rehabilitation from such injuries is very difficult in a patient with Alzheimer's disease, and falls should be prevented by any means possible.

Increasing problems with toileting, incontinence, and adult diapers

As the disease progresses the patient becomes less and less aware of when they need to go to the bathroom. While in the middle stages this can probably be managed by taking the patient to the bathroom every couple of hours with only the occasional episode of incontinence, at this stage of the disease more drastic measures need to be taken. Accordingly, let me introduce you and your patient to the wonderful world of adult disposable diapers, sold as Depends or similar charmingly-named products. Many patients will resist this idea at first, and will initially refuse to wear such garments, either at night or in the daytime. But as the experience of wetting themselves or soiling themselves becomes more frequent, and the clean-up process becomes more burdensome and unpleasant, most patients eventually accept the need to wear such garments. While this lightens the burden of the caregiver somewhat, there is still the huge task of keeping the patient clean and dry at all times. If you have had some experience diapering babies, you may be somewhat prepared for this task. If not, it is just something that you will have to learn to do. When the physical cleaning must first be done, both men and women can become embarrassed at being cleaned up after removal of the protective undergarment. This is especially difficult when the patient no longer recognizes the caregiver. Many a female patient has said, "You can't do this to me, I am a married woman." Many a male caregiver, who may have never diapered a baby, may find this task particularly unappealing. The part of the body they once worshipped only for sexual congress now becomes simply a work area. The daughter of a patient with Alzheimer's disease had the challenging experience of being a caregiver at somewhat of a distance: her mother, in the early stages of her disease, had begun an intimate relationship with a widower, and eventually moved in with him. The widower, John, was very fond of the mother and insisted that he would take care of "my baby," as he called her. One day the daughter was faced with a startling situation. She wrote up this experience in the following story, which she called "Afternoon Surprise:"

My mother has Alzheimer's disease, poor thing. She was diagnosed about a year ago after she got lost driving to the beauty parlor. She had only been going there once a week for the last three years, or as long as she had lived with John. But that is another story. I took her to my own doctor and told him I was concerned about her memory, and that she had gotten lost the other day. The doctor asked her the date and gave her three words to remember, and she couldn't do either one. So he sent her to have an MRI done, and afterwards told me and her that she had "a memory problem." He didn't use the "A" word with her, but I knew. He told her he was going to put her on some medicine, Aricept that would help her memory, to which she said "okay." That was a year ago.

Today I came to pick her up to go grocery shopping, which she likes to do with me. Boy, did I get a surprise! As I drove up to John's house, I saw she was sitting on the front porch. In front of her there were eight suitcases all lined up: her two carry-on bags that she used to take on trips with her; an old cardboard suitcase that was beginning to come apart; and five other cases that were more or less just moving boxes with string wrapped around them, to make them look like suitcases.

"What's up, Mom?" I said.

"I guess John doesn't want me anymore."

Just then John came out the front door, looking down, not looking me in the eye. I said: "What's up, John?"

And he said, "Joanne, you're going to have to take your mom home with you. I just can't take it anymore. I'm sorry."

They had lived together for three years. He really seemed to care about her. He used to go to the doctor with her, and ask him questions about what he was supposed to do.

The doctor had told me: "When she becomes incontinent, he may not be able to handle it anymore." So I guess I had been warned. I put my

*arms around Mom, and she hers around me, and
we both had a good cry. Then I loaded six of the
suitcases in the back of my station wagon, and put
the two carry-on bags on the back seat. Then we
both got in my car and drove off.*

This story illustrates how difficult if may be for a male
caregiver to provide incontinence care to his wife. In the
case above where the "significant other" had known the
patient for only a short period of time, the man was unable
to cope with this task in an ongoing way. Clearly, there was
pain on both sides, and the daughter did what she had to do.
She stepped in to fill the void.

What you need to consider when your loved one needs to be placed in a facility

As the burdens of caregiving increase, you will need to
face what may be one of the most agonizing decisions you
will ever make: when to place your loved one into a care
facility especially designed for memory-impaired persons.
As the person you are caring for becomes less and less able
to cooperate with you, in terms of dressing and bathing but
especially in terms of getting to the bathroom on time, it will
be best to consider finding a place where more than one
person will be able to provide the needed care, i.e. admission
to either an assisted living facility or a specialized memory
care unit in a nursing home. It will simply not be possible
for one person to physically care for someone who can no
longer cooperate actively with the caregiver. Moreover, you
should not have to make this decision by yourself, but
should do so in concert with the patient's doctor who can
advise you when it the time is right to implement this
decision.

Please be assured that in making this decision, you are in no way abandoning the care of your loved one. You will still be in charge, although perhaps somewhat at arm's length, of assuring the proper care is provided. Please be further assured that at this stage of the disease, care in a specialized facility will be the absolutely best thing that you can do for the affected person.

What type of facility is available to provide care for your loved one?

Fortunately there are now a number of types of facilities that are able to provide excellent care for your loved one. These include Alzheimer's Assisted Living Facilities and specialized Memory Care Units in nursing homes. The critical component of these units is not the label "Alzheimer's Care Unit" or "Memory-Impaired Unit" but whether the staff of such a unit has undergone *special training in caring for memory-impaired individuals.* An Alzheimer's Assisted Living Facility will be appropriate for individuals who can still provide basic self-care activities, such as eating, dressing, and getting in and out of bed, for themselves. A Memory-Impaired Unit in a nursing home will be appropriate for individuals who now need assistance in feeding, dressing, and getting in and out of bed for themselves. One suggestion is that you visit such units with a friend or a relative, for support, and so that you can share thoughts and impressions about the facility.

I recommend that you plan to visit several such units *before* the need for placement of your loved one becomes necessary. Thereby you will be able to choose in advance the kind of facility that meets your requirements: a clean, home-like atmosphere, with staff trained to assist memory-impaired patients with whatever activities they require. Then, when the time comes to place your loved one in a facility, you will be assured that you have made the best choice possible.

"But I promised my mother I would never put her in a nursing home."

Many times I have heard a caregiver utter this phrase, in complete agony, as he or she is considering the need to find a facility for ongoing care of their loved one, whether it is a wife, a husband, or a mother. While I would like to advise all caregivers not to make such promises to their loved ones, it is often too late, and such promises have been made. Here is the solution: in these cases I will counsel with the caregiver to the effect that they made that promise to their loved one when they were an entirely different person. They are now making the decision for a person who is in need of care and in a very different mental and physical state than was the person to whom they made that promise.

One husband, Harry, confided in me how he felt about admitting his wife Mary to a specialized memory care unit in a nursing home. He said: "When she no longer knows that she and I belong together, then I'll be able to let her go." Harry continued to visit his wife in the nursing home every day until she finally passed away.

Keep in mind that the old image of a nursing home that you or your loved one may have once had as a place with the smell of urine, minimal attention to the needs of the patients, and a staff untrained in dealing with memory-impaired patients, is no longer true. Today you will be able to find a nursing home that specializes in caring for memory-impaired persons in a home-like atmosphere, with a full range of activities geared to the abilities of its residents, a caring staff that are willing and able to speak with you, the responsible caregiver, whenever you need to do so. You may need to visit several possible facilities to find the right one for your loved one, but it is possible to do so now. Importantly, ask members of your caregiver support group for names and ideas of where to look, based on their experience with such places.

Not that it is ever easy to have to place a loved one into a facility. Here is how one caregiver described his agony at seeing his wife in the care facility, with shrinking abilities, with a fading personality, and her ability to recognize him as her husband becoming a sometime thing. He wrote:

TRY TO IMAGINE:

While you are out of town, lightning strikes your house and it burns to the ground. This is the home you've loved and lived in for decades. Your neighbor tells you the news and you come right back.

You park out front and there is the location and the lot and the foundation, but the structure that made it a house is gone and is just a smoldering bed of gray ashes. All the possessions, valuables, heirlooms, photos, memorabilia and memories that made it home are gone too and lie in those ashes.

Your emotions well up as you contemplate what you have lost. It's beyond your comprehension, you can't grasp it all at once, and you are left hanging. And it is all so clearly final.

That's what it is like when I visit my wife, in the care facility where what remains of her resides. The familiar foundation is there, but the intellect, the spirit, the emotion, the responses, that had made her a loving wife for so many years, are gone. And it is all so clearly final.

The role of hospice care in the late stages of Alzheimer's disease

There is one other type of care that you may wish to consider for your loved one in the late stages of Alzheimer's disease. When someone has reached the stage in medical care where full recovery is not possible, hospice care can be instituted. Hospice care provides end of life care which is devoted to making the person comfortable. Those who are experiencing pain can be kept pain-free with a regimen of powerful medication, without concern about becoming addicted. Hospice care is perhaps most commonly used for patients with disseminated cancer. But it can also be used for someone in the late stages of Alzheimer's disease, heart disease, chronic obstructive pulmonary disease, or any other terminal condition. Care is provided either in the patient's own home or in a home-like setting, but it can also be provided for someone in a nursing home. Psychological comfort and communication with family members and friends is emphasized. Importantly, hospice care is provided at no additional cost as a regular Medicare or Medicaid benefit.

Hospice services may include ongoing care by physicians, nurses, social workers or mental health specialists. An important aspect of hospice care is that trained volunteers make up a significant part of the hospice personnel. Such volunteers can provide emotional support, companionship, run errands or provide transportation.

"There are tears in things"

In these last three chapters we have discussed the various stages of Alzheimer's disease as though they were clearly separate and distinct from one another. The fact is, however, and you will have noticed this as you have lived with this disease, that these stages flow into one another in a continuing process. But at every stage there is one constant feature: sadness and tears. Virgil, the Roman poet, said in the Aeneid: "*sunt lacrima rerum,*' which translated means "there are tears in things." Indeed there "are tears in things that forever haunt the fragile human heart" throughout all the stages of Alzheimer's disease. That is why this book was written, and that is why researchers everywhere are striving to create "a world without Alzheimer's disease. Until that day, caregivers like you are helping to make living with Alzheimer's humane and possible.

Chapter Summary

1. **Memory problems are now much worse.**

2. **Verbal communications are now quite limited.**

3. **Behavioral problems become more prominent.**

4. **Increasing problems with toileting, incontinence, and adult diapers.**

5. **Consider what you need to do when your loved one has to be placed in a facility.**

6. **Become familiar with the kinds of facilities in your community that can provide care for memory-impaired persons.**

7. **"But I promised my mother I would never put her in a nursing home." Remember you are now dealing with an entirely different person.**

8. **Understand the role of hospice care in the late stages of Alzheimer's disease.**

9. **Yes, there are tears in things.**

Chapter Twelve

Caregivers Need Care, Too

Caregivers have many unmet needs

For the last several chapters we have been speaking about what the patient needs from the caregiver. Now it is time to turn to your needs -- you, the caregiver. Early on in my work with caregivers I was struck by the fact that for all that caregivers gave, they themselves had many unmet needs. In short, I realized that *caregivers need care, too.* Caregivers need: information about the illness they are dealing with and its course; they need emotional support and recognition for the many contributions they are making. They also need knowledge about community resources, about legal and financial issues, and practical information for coping with troublesome behaviors. They also need to understand the nature of the caregiver role, and how to protect their own well-being and self-esteem.

Join an Alzheimer's caregiver support group

As I've already said in discussing the early stages of Alzheimer's disease, one of the best things that a caregiver can do is to *join an Alzheimer's caregiver support group*. In a caregiver support group you will meet regularly with perhaps a dozen other caregivers with whom you can share and from whom you can learn any number of techniques which you can immediately apply for dealing with issues as they arise. Such caregiver support groups are often organized by memory disorder clinics associated with major hospitals or a medical school. Frequently, one of the members of the professional staff, either a nurse, a doctor, or a social worker, serve as facilitators of such support groups. The leader of such a group needs to fully understand Alzheimer's disease and the role of caregivers, as well as having skills in group process. Most caregivers feel that participation in a caregiver support group has a profound healing effect. They realize that they are not alone, that other caregivers are going through similar experiences, and that they are participating in a caring community. Later on they will also benefit from the fact that, from time to time, they will be able to make a contribution to their fellow caregivers, by sharing an insight or a new technique that they have learned or created. Moreover, they will find that they can bring up any kind of question at all that is troubling them without fear of disapproval or fear of not being taken seriously. A caregiver group is a *safe house.*

Wherein lies the genius, the magic, of caregiver support groups?

This is not an easy question to answer, but caregivers have told me over and over that the magic is real, that is has a healing effect, and that nothing that happens in the process of caregiving is off limits for discussion in a caregiver group. More often than not, any new problem that crops up for someone has already been dealt with by someone else. And even if that is not the case members of the caregiver group will often work out a possible solution to the new problem. It really functions as a mastermind group to address with the ever-changing problems caregivers face. And information about new opportunities, such as participation in a promising clinical study, will spread like wildfire among the group. Often have I heard from caregivers that did not have the advantage of belonging to a caregiver group, how they feel they missed out on a vital life-line. And one of the most valuable things that you can do for someone new to caregiving is to persuade them to find and join such a group.

To be sure, not all groups will meet the needs of everyone in the group. One experienced caregiver advises that you *try more than one* group, either to learn some things from one group and some from another, or to keep trying new groups until you find one that really "fits."

Of course, caregiver support groups are made up of all kinds of people: men and women, spouses and ex-spouses, sons and daughters, sons-in-law and daughters-in-law, each bringing a somewhat differing point of view to the caregiver experience. Be assured, you can learn something from each of them. Each of them, in turn, can learn something from you. You might be interested in hearing how one member of a caregiver support group saw the process. He wrote the following about Alzheimer's caregiver support groups:

> *I have attended numerous meetings of support groups for people caring for family members suffering from senile dementia of the Alzheimer type. During this time I have gradually become aware of an interesting feature. There is a substantial difference between those persons caring for a spouse and those caring for a parent. The two groups have significantly different views of the problems, the ways to cope with them, the outcomes they hope for and especially in their interactions with the patient. When more than one child is involved in a parent's care the differences are even greater and more obvious.*

I conclude that the basic reason for this is that when a couple marries they tend to grow closer to each other, while as children grow and mature they tend to grow apart from their parents. There is a rather stable period of decades from the time the children become independent until the parents succumb to old age. Then, a whole new relationship starts to develop as the child grows closer to the parent but now with the care giving roles reversed. This new relationship is foreign to both parties and very difficult for each to understand and accept. Meanwhile, the spouses continue caring for each other as before, to the extent that each is still able.

This situation is entirely natural and normal. It is neither right nor wrong. It is simply a fact of life. Now that I have finally recognized it and brought it into focus, it has helped me to understand and evaluate the remarks and feelings of the other members of the support groups and has influenced the way I now respond to those members.

John W. Luce 2008 June 9

There are many lessons that you can learn from participating in caregiver support groups. One of the most important of these is the following:

Learn to Share the Burden of Care

Despite what you may have believed at the outset, it is possible, no, *it is necessary, to share the burden of care* for someone with Alzheimer's disease. It is quite natural that you may want to do everything yourself, perhaps because you fear that no one else will be able to do as good a job of caring for your loved one as you can. And you are right. However, there will be times and parts of the job that it will be wise for you to share with someone else or to delegate to someone else. Fear not, you will remain in charge of all that will be done for your loved one. To illustrate that you are not alone in hesitating to delegate any part of the caregiving task to someone else, let me tell you about one such situation, the case of Manuel and Cathy:

Manuel was a successful businessman, community leader, and philanthropist. He and his wife, Cathy, were very close. They went everywhere together. At age 70, Cathy began to repeat herself incessantly; she often misplaced her keys, lost her checkbook, and needed to be reminded about appointments she had. At first, Manuel tried to rationalize Cathy's forgetfulness and hide his concern about her from friends and family members. He didn't want to believe that she could possibly be developing Alzheimer's disease. However, as her symptoms continued to worsen, he became sufficiently concerned that he sought professional help. Cathy was evaluated, and doctors told Manuel that she did indeed have Alzheimer's disease. Cathy was quickly started on treatment. Early on, her doctor advised Manuel that he should consider seeking help with caring for his wife, but he insisted that he would be the only one to look after her. Both he and Cathy were very private people, and neither one wanted to accept the idea of a stranger coming into their home. As Cathy became more and more impaired, and Manuel had to do more and more for her, he became increasingly depressed and tired, but he still refused to get any help with his caregiving duties. Cathy got up several times during the night, was agitated, and Manuel got very little sleep. Still, he insisted that he do everything for her, and that no one else could care for Cathy as well as he could. Then, within 24 hours, two things happened: Cathy got up in the middle of the night and fell in the bathroom, injuring her chest and her head. Manuel himself injured his back trying to lift her from the bathroom floor. He finally called his daughter and allowed her to bring in live-in help for both of them. A few weeks later he confessed to Cathy's doctor, "I'm so relieved we have help now. I should have listened to your advice a lot sooner.

Learn to share the burden of care sooner rather than later.

The take-home lesson from the story of Manuel and Cathy is that you need to learn to share the burden of care sooner rather than later. This is for your benefit as well as for the benefit of your loved one. If you can introduce additional help at a stage when your loved one can still form new relationships easily, it will ease the need to accept additional help later on in the course of the illness. It really does take a team of caregivers to provide all the help that is needed. Have no fear; you will always be the head of the team, the coach to help others help you. Your life and that of your loved one will be richer for it. There will be less pain, less grief, less isolation. So allow yourself to be helped! One of the most powerful phrases in the English or any other language is: "I need your help." Nobody ever minds being asked to help.

If you think I am going overboard in insisting on planning and on sharing the burden of care, here is a quick reality check.

If you think I have gone overboard in insisting that you seek and get help early on in your caregiver experience, let me tell you the stark reality of why I am being both insistent and persistent on this point: caregivers are not invulnerable. Without help they can become discouraged, depressed, or suffer burn-out; they can begin to neglect their own care or the care of their patient. Some totally distressed caregivers can even become abusive to their loved ones when they feel at the end of their rope. You don't want to be among them. Caregiver help helps prevent such outcomes.

But there is yet another reason for careful planning and for assuring that someone else can provide some of the care needed: It is possible that you may die before your loved one. You may have an accident, develop an unforeseen medical problem, or fall victim to a natural or civil disaster. Planning ahead and sharing the burden of care will guard against the consequences of such outcomes as well.

Daycare

As part of my advice to you as a caregiver to "share the burden of care," I recommend that you consider having your loved one participate in an adult daycare program for memory-impaired people. This is particularly relevant during the long months and years when the patient is in the middle stages of the disease. In the early stages of the disease the patient may resent going to a daycare program, possibly seeing it as demeaning. In the late stages they may not be able to participate in the many activities offered by daycare programs. These can include socializing, reminiscing, dancing, simple exercise activities, listening to music or sing-alongs, or watching movie comedies. The socialization with staff and with other patients that goes on in daycare programs is also of great benefit to the patients. And not unimportant, it gives you, the caregiver, time for yourself for those hours each day that the patient participates. Some programs are open up to five times a week, or even on weekends. Use those times to attend to your own needs, go to the beauty parlor or the barbershop, play golf, go to the doctor, socialize with your friends, or just have fun. It is allowed! Or do whatever will contribute to your own health and happiness. You will return to caregiving so much more refreshed and restored. The patient, too, will benefit greatly from having been with someone else as well, and that is no knock on your contribution.

The cost of participating in daycare programs is generally low, as it is either supported by public programs, or can be arranged on a sliding scale basis, according to your financial status. Adult day care programs may be operated by memory disorder clinics, councils on aging, assisted living facilities, or even as freestanding not-for profit operations.

Respite care

While having your patient attend adult daycare will give you short periods of relief, certain events may crop up in your life that require a longer period of time away from caregiving: the wedding of an adult child or other relative, graduation from college, a family reunion, or even an elective medical procedure. Maybe you would like to have a face-lift done, or you might just need a much deserved, honest-to-goodness vacation. For occasions like this, I recommend that you consider placing your patient into a *respite care program*. Respite care for a week or two, sometimes even up to three weeks, is provided by a number of enlightened assisted living facilities or nursing homes that operate special memory care units. Your loved one will receive excellent care there while you are away. And you both will look forward to a welcome reunion. Sometimes this can also serve as a preview of the kind of care your patient might receive at such a facility, as you may eventually have to consider placing your loved into such care. But I would keep this part of your purpose to yourself for now.

The cost of respite care programs also is generally affordable, or it may be supported by charitable organizations. The Alzheimer's Association conducts such programs in many communities, as do some nursing homes, in part as a marketing tool. The Veterans Administration also offers respite care to eligible veterans. Again, cost should not stand in the way of using this highly beneficial service.

Start a caregiver exchange program

Another "invention" that I have seen some caregivers create is a caregiver exchange program. You trade off caregiving for your patient with another caregiver, each of you in turn taking care of two patients who are compatible with one another. Again, such exchanges will benefit both participating caregivers and patients.

Take your loved one on a cruise.

Cruises for a few days, up to two weeks, are almost ideal ways of giving both you and your loved one a break. This should be done in the early or middle stages of the disease, so that your loved can still maneuver about, enjoy the sights and sounds, the entertainment, and all the other activities, and Oh, the meals, under your supervision. Careful planning needs to go into this to assure that the cruise will not be too demanding on either one of you, but the self-contained environment of a cruise can be very enjoyable for both patient and caregiver. Or you might want to take another caregiver, a relative or friend, along to share caregiving duties. And then tell your caregiver support group about the experience! I bet you will get a round of applause, and a little bit of envy.

Recruit and deputize an assistant caregiver

At any stage of the disease you could implement a plan to train somebody else as a deputy caregiver. This could be a sibling who doesn't have time for caregiving all the time, a friend, someone from your church or other social group, or your spouse (if he is not the patient as well). You could also hire someone, if there is not someone in your social circle who could provide the occasional caregiver break to you. Consider hiring a college student, or a retired person who could use the extra money, or use your imagination or the combined imagination of your caregiver support group to come up with another likely candidate for a deputy caregiver. Your loved one will surely come to enjoy the change of pace, even if they might not be happy about it immediately. I certainly have seen this strategy work very effectively in many cases, and in many differing ways.

If you heed all my advice, and that based on the experience of other caregivers, you will soon be mastering the caregiver experience.

All of the ways I have described for providing care for the caregiver and for sharing the burden of care are designed to maintain your health, your mental health, your strength, and your zest for caregiving.

Chapter Summary

1. Caregivers have many unmet needs.

2. Join an Alzheimer's caregiver support group.

3. Come to understand wherein lies the genius, the magic, of caregiver groups.

4. Learn to share the burden of care.

5. Learn to share the burden of care sooner rather than later.

6. If you think I am going overboard in insisting on planning and sharing the burden of care, here is a quick reality check.

7. Make use of adult daycare for your loved one.

8. Learn about respite care, for yourself, and for your loved one.

9. Or start a caregiver exchange program.

10. Or go on a cruise with your loved one.

11. Recruit and deputize an assistant caregiver.

12. Then, if you heed my advice, you will soon be mastering the caregiver experience.

Chapter Thirteen

When Your Loved One Dies

Your long journey of caregiving has ended

One insightful person describing the experience of someone caring for an Alzheimer's patient called it "The Long Good-Bye." Undoubtedly, over the course of the months and years that you have seen your loved one lose characteristics and abilities that you once cherished, you have in fact been saying good-bye to him or her right along. However, when the time comes that your loved one actually dies, you will be surprised that you will be faced with a new kind of loss, a new kind of grief, based on the finality of that moment. As the gentleman whom we quoted earlier on said, "but I still know her," you won't be saying even that anymore. There will be no one to visit, no one's hand to hold, and no one's brow to stroke. The loss will be quite devastating all over again.

Along with grief, you may also experience a sense of relief

If you are like most people, it is likely that, along with your grief, you will also feel a certain amount of relief over the fact that your loved one is now at peace, and that your task as a caregiver has come to an end. That is as it should be. Some people feel guilty for having this sense of relief. But this relief is entirely normal, and not anything for which you should feel guilty. You can be proud for all that you have done, knowing that you made a positive difference in the life of your loved one, at a time when they most needed it. You have been a good and faithful servant, and it is now time for this chapter of your life to end, to close the book on caregiving, to be grateful for having been able to be of service in ways that mattered profoundly. It is now time to celebrate the life that has been laid to rest, and the affection and the commitment between you and your loved one, the likes of which will not come again. It is finished.

Of course, life goes on, even when it doesn't. You will be occupied with funeral arrangements, obituaries to be published, memorial services to be arranged, death certificates to be obtained, and to be distributed to all those requiring them: important things to accomplish, but nothing compared to the relationship you once had. It will be a time of remembering and a time of grieving. Before all that comes to be, however, there is one decision you may need to make before all the others: whether to have a brain autopsy conducted on your loved one.

Should you consider having a brain autopsy done?

In order to have a brain autopsy done you need to plan well ahead. Permission forms need to be signed and arrangements made with a brain bank in your area. But there are very good reasons for having an autopsy performed at the time your loved one dies: 1. to confirm the diagnosis; and 2. to contribute to research on Alzheimer's disease. In general it is necessary to have the brain collected for examination as quickly as possible, usually within two to four hours after death. This can be done through whoever will be handling funeral arrangements. It will not disturb the physical appearance of your loved one. Or, it may be something that you and your loved had long ago decided you will not pursue. If you do proceed you will be informed whether the physical hallmarks of Alzheimer's disease were in fact present in the brain of your loved one. You will be told to what extent amyloid plaques and fibrillary tangles were found. This will give you closure that you were in fact dealing with Alzheimer's disease. Brain tissue can then be used in research to find a solution to this most vexing and puzzling disease. If you follow this course, you and your loved one will have contributed to what is our highest goal for the future: *a world without Alzheimer's disease.*

You will now gather around you those who are dear to you

This is the time to gather around you those who are dearest to you. They will share in your grief and they will share in your remembering the one you have lost. Memories of the one you loved will remain forever, even though their memory disappeared tragically before its time. No one else could have done what you have done. All those who understand what you have done will be grateful to you forever.

Chapter Summary

1. **Your long journey of caregiving has ended.**

2. **There is no need to have feelings of guilt over the sense of relief you feel.**

3. **Should you consider having a brain autopsy performed on your loved one? If so, you need to plan for it well ahead.**

4. **Now you will gather around you those who are dear to you.**

5. **All those who understand what you have done will be grateful to you forever.**

Chapter Fourteen

When Your Caregiving Days Are Over

Your days as a caregiver are now over

When your career as a caregiver of an Alzheimer's patient has ended, it is time to resume your own life. Looking back on this time will be instructive: you will have learned many new skills; you will have been challenged to be creative in ways never demanded before; you will have experienced many triumphs in dealing with crises and extreme difficulties. As a result, you are now ready for anything. But wait! Before charging ahead with your new life, there is something else that you must first do:

Take time to recover from the exhaustion that you, like most caregivers, will have experienced.

At the end of your caregiving you may discover that you, like many other caregivers, are profoundly exhausted, or "bone-tired," emotionally and physically, as more than one caregiver has confided to me. You will want to take time to replenish your resources, to catch up on sleep, to resume your exercise program, to have meals on a regular schedule, yes, even to indulge yourself a little. You will want to tell your friends and your family that you are "back" and that you want to be re-included in their activities. How long will that take? Well, it might be weeks or months, depending on what you do and on what support you get from others. A number of caregivers I know have continued to attend their support groups. There they continue to receive the love and affection of other group members, but there they can also share the fact that they themselves are now "recovering," and that soon they will be ready to resume a new and a full life that might include anything. And what might that "anything" be for you?

You could apply your knowledge of caregiving to help other caregivers

You might apply the knowledge you have gained to help other people struggling with caregiving tasks. Certainly there is a great need for this; and you would be highly rewarded for teaching others what you have learned during your long career as a caregiver. Or you might become a fund-raiser for Alzheimer's disease research, since you know well that further progress in this area is desperately needed.

You could write a book about your caregiving experience

Or you could even write a book about your caregiver experience. You would have much to share, and many would be grateful for what they could learn from your journey. An even more interesting variation on this theme might be for you to *write a book about the person for whom you provided care*. Now there is an idea!

Or you may wish to turn in an entirely new direction

On the other hand, you may wish to turn completely away from having any further dealings with this disease, and pursue all those activities that had to be back-burnered during your caregiving career. This might include reconnecting with other family members, friends whom you may have had to neglect while caregiving, or to pursue other creative or spiritual activities. A long and a long-delayed vacation would certainly be something you deserve, and which you can now enjoy.

You are a modern day hero. Thank you, thank you, and thank you.

Whatever activities you may wish to undertake, you will be able to do so with greater skills and confidence than you ever had before. You have grown, you have matured, and you have extended your capabilities to where there is nothing that you cannot do. Nothing could be more difficult than what you have been through. I personally believe that you as a caregiver of someone with Alzheimer's disease have truly been a modern hero or heroine. Congratulations! Well done! You have every reason to be truly proud of yourself. The power of your shining example will be there for others to follow. Thank you. Thank you. And I say this on behalf of all the patients who can no longer say it themselves.

Chapter Summary

1. **Your days as a caregiver are now over.**

2. **Take time to recover from the exhaustion that you, like most caregivers, will have experienced.**

3. **You could apply your knowledge of caregiving to help other caregivers.**

4. **You could write a book about your caregiving experience.**

5. **Or you wish to turn in an entirely new direction.**

6. **You are a modern day hero. Thank you, thank you, and thank you.**

Chapter Fifteen

Post-Script

Having finished the manuscript for this book, I felt the need to re-connect with some of the most successful caregivers I had come to know over a period of some thirty years. After some reflection on what I, and by extension, what you could still learn from them, I called together a group of seven experienced caregivers, two men, and five women, for a Sunday afternoon get-together to reflect on their caregiver experiences and to harvest lessons that could be learned. It was a very moving experience for all of us. We felt very close to one another, and I believe we all felt privileged to be with one another. They each had read the manuscript sometime during the preceding week, and each in turn expressed the feeling that they wished such a book had been available to them when they began their caregiving experience. Nearly everyone that afternoon said they wanted to make copies of the book available to their friends who were just now facing a similar challenge.

I asked each of them to respond to five simple questions. Each gave very thoughtful but widely differing responses to these questions. I thought you, the reader, might be enlightened by what they had to say. I first tried to summarize their responses, but came to feel that that could not do full justice to their wisdom and their creativity. Accordingly, I am going to let each of them speak for themselves.

So here are the five questions, and the responses of each of my seven caregiver friends:

1. **What was the hardest thing about your caregiving experience?**

2. **What was the most rewarding thing about it?**

3. **What was the best advice anyone gave you about your caregiving tasks?**

4. **What advice would give someone just starting on their caregiver experience?**

5. **What other specific topics should be included in such a book?**

Here are their answers:

Question One: What was the hardest thing about your caregiver experience?

Helen: "That was almost thirty years ago. Nobody had ever heard of Alzheimer's disease. It was hard because you feel so isolated. It really separates your friends from your acquaintances. It as exhausting, it was draining. Even when you are out with friends, it sits on your shoulder. And, of course, your heart is broken."

John: "Sending my wife to a facility, even though it was the best thing for both of us."

Pat G.: "The only thing that was available then was a nursing home. And they were really still very understaffed then. The other thing that was hard for me was to see my Mom let the nurses do things for her that she wouldn't let me do."

Ed: "Seeing the gradual decline of my mother-in-law over a number of years."

Pat B.: "The loneliness. The isolation that I felt and that he felt, too. I wondered if people felt the disease was contagious. They would come near him, they wouldn't touch him. Only one person, a close friend, came to greet us and touch him. Your friends stop talking to you. They stay away."

Shirley: "Not having my Mom to talk to any more. And the role change when I was suddenly the parent and she the child."

Dolly: "Putting my Mom in the Assisted Living Unit. It was terrible to see her distress and confusion. That really got to me, and it still does." (she breaks into tears)

Question Two: What was the most rewarding aspect of your caregiver experience?

Helen: "Was there anything rewarding? It was very hard. I guess I was glad that I finally got some help. I finally understood what to expect next. That was a blessing. I felt compelled to do this since he had taken such wonderful care of me and the children for so many years."

John: "I didn't find it very rewarding. But I felt rewarded by being able to help others in the support group based on what I had learned."

Pat G.: "It taught me about Alzheimer's disease. It was also very rewarding that my Mom knew me until she died. I always felt she knew me, even when she thought I was her mother."

Ed: "It prompted me to assist one of the first caregiver support groups in the area to become an Alzheimer's Association Chapter, which I then ran for six years."

Pat B.:   "During the time it didn't seem very rewarding. But looking back, it was a real education. I learned humility. I learned to arrange life so that it suited both of us, not just me alone. I kept taking him to our place of business, and I kept him so well dressed and groomed that many people didn't even know he was ill."

Shirley: "Yes, there were many rewards, and I made the commitment to it, even though I had to retire twelve years early from my job. I loved finding little things to do with her, like reciting nursery rhymes that she remembered or singing songs together. "You Are My Sunshine" was her favorite, and we sang it everywhere, in the doctor's office, or in the car, and I don't care that people stared at us."

Dolly: "The little things. That I could still spend quality time with my Mom. Yes, I was glad that I was available to help. I knew she had always loved puzzles. So would find or invent simple puzzles that she could still do, and we would do them together."

Question Three: What was the best advice anyone gave you about your caregiver tasks?

Helen: "You can't argue with them."

John: "The doctor was worried about my health condition. So he told me to take her to a facility. What was surprising was that she settled in fairly well, without a lot of distress on her part. She accepted it."

Pat G.:   "Bringing familiar things to her room at the facility. I was told to get help, to get out of the "I can do it alone" mode. And to get help when the patient can still form a relationship with other helpers."

Ed: "There will be conflict, and misbehavior. But it will not be willful on the part of the patient. It is the disease. Don't do battle with the person; you may just have to walk away for a bit."

Pat B.:   "Take care of yourself! The patient could outlive you if you died or were to fall apart."

Shirley: "Not a lot of advice was available. I had to go through a lot of trial and error. You need so much *patience!* And what works today will not necessarily work tomorrow. You have to keep adapting. When my Mom would not take a bath, I said "We are going to make you queen for a day. Her name was Elizabeth, and I would call her Queen Elizabeth, and we would go to the spa in our own bathroom, and she would have her hair done and look really beautiful. That way she took a bath with happiness and pleasure."

Dolly: "Go to a caregiver conference! It really helped. I learned so much in one day. I also learned about going to 'post-graduation' caregiver support groups."

Question Four: What advice would you give someone just starting out on their caregiver experience?

Helen: "Find a support group, and get help early. If there is a university in your community, see what it has to offer."

John: "You've got to belong to a caregiver group. You might even join more than one, because they have different things to offer. When you can't take care of the person any longer, it is not a reflection on you."

Pat G.:   "Get an elder law attorney early while you both can still participate."

Ed: "Begin the organization of family resources as soon as the diagnosis has been made. Identify necessary and qualified medical and legal support services. Develop and implement a checklist to follow. Include other family members from the beginning."

Pat B.:   "For our fiftieth anniversary we had a big celebration. A lot of people came and he just sat there. That evening he didn't remember a thing. But it is still important to do those kinds of things for the person. It was also important to me and to my daughter."

Dolly: "Pass on the advice that you get. Learn extreme patience. Remember you are not dealing with your Mom or Dad, but with a new person who has the illness."

Question Five: What other topics should be included in a book on caregiving in Alzheimer's disease?

Helen: "There IS life after Alzheimer's!"

John: "That there are other forms of dementia, such as vascular dementia, Lewy Body Disease, and normal pressure hydrocephalus."

Pat G.:   "The need for long-distance caregiving."

Ed G.:   "Right at the beginning, when the diagnosis is first made, there is the need for power of attorney and for a healthcare surrogate. Make sure that the larger family understands what is needed and why it is needed."

Pat B.:   "Make this book available to any new caregiver, even those caring for people with other diseases. They can learn from the Alzheimer's caregiver experience."

Shirley: "Tell people where they can find information. Also, to know about adult protective services for people who don't have a caregiver."

Dolly: "This book needs to go to doctors as well as caregivers, and to relatives and friends, so that they understand what the caregiver is going through."

Wow! There was a whole lot of wisdom, and a huge amount of emotion in that room that Sunday afternoon. There was not a dry eye in the house. I hope that I have done justice to all the participants. But here is an idea: when you want to fully understand what you have been going through while caring for your loved one with Alzheimer's disease, call a group of your former support group members together and share your remembrances. And be sure to have plenty of Kleenex on hand.

Appendix

Caregiver Nuggets

In this section I am going to discuss a number of topics related to the care of an Alzheimer's patient which may only be relevant to some patients, or which I didn't feel deserved a full chapter. Please, browse through this section and read those topics which strike you as relevant to your loved one. Or you may return to some of these topics, if and when they become relevant to your situation at some point later on in your caregiving.

Ability to make a will

In the early stages of Alzheimer's disease someone with Alzheimer's disease is still capable of making a will or of amending an existing will. This is so because the legal requirements for making a valid will are relatively simple. The person making a will must understand that they are making a will and that the making of a will generally relates to the distribution of the property and valuables after they have died; the person must also know and understand what is called in legal terms "the natural objects of their bounty." That means the person must be aware who his family members and close friends are, and whether the person wishes to bequeath part of all of their possessions to those persons. The third requirement is that the person understands the nature and location of their properties, valuables, and so on.

However, because wills of persons with Alzheimer's disease are often contested on the basis that the person no longer understood what they were doing, or that undue influence was used to obtain a specific will provision, the fact and circumstances of a will being drafted or amended by a person in the early stages of the disease should specify how and where the will was made, who was in attendance, that there was medical certification that the person was still capable of making a such a will or amendment to the will. After the early stages of Alzheimer's diseases, it is advisable that no new wills be created and that no significant amendments to an existing will be made. This also reinforces the general advice that wills be made and amended in a timely fashion, when all physical and mental capabilities are still intact.

Adult Protective Services

People with Alzheimer's disease who are living alone, or who don't have any family member or close friend who could provide care, should be referred to social service agencies. Primary responders, such as police and firefighters need to be made aware of the problem of Alzheimer's patients who have no one to care for them. The patient can be referred or admitted to special care assisted living facilities where much of the services that would be provided by a family caregiver can be provided by a professional trained caregiver.

Alzheimer's Association

The Alzheimer's Association is the largest nation-wide advocacy organization in support of individuals affected by Alzheimer's disease. It provides information about diagnostic and treatment services, caregiver support services, description of the disease, and other issues. It has local chapters in many communities throughout the United States. The Association has a significant lobbying arm which seeks to influence federal legislation related to Alzheimer's disease research and services. 24/7 telephone helpline: 1-800-272-3900. Internet contact: alz.org.

Area Agencies on Aging

Area Agencies on Aging are federally funded community organizations designed to assist elderly persons in finding health, social, respite, and other services. They can also help you find volunteer opportunities, meal service sites, and senior centers as well as respite care programs. Every sizeable community has one or is served by one. They can be found in your local phone books under a listing of federal government agencies, or through the National Eldercare Locator. Look up Eldercare Locator in this Section.

Assisted Living Facilities

Assisted Living Facilities, or ALFs, are residential facilities that provide basic food and shelter for people who are no longer able to provide these for themselves. Care in ALFs is not covered by Medicare or Medicaid, but is specifically covered by some long term care insurance policies. Some ALFs only provide assistance with basic self-care while others may additionally provide medication administration and medical monitoring, such as blood pressure measurements or blood sugar testing.

Caregiver seminars

At the University of South Florida we began to conduct caregiver training seminars for individuals engaged at all levels of caregiving for an Alzheimer's patient. These are day-long seminars in which all aspects of Alzheimer's disease and all aspects of caregiving are discussed by a series of experts on medical, social, legal and financial aspects of caregiving. Caregivers are encouraged to ask questions and present problems to these experts for solution. These caregiver seminars have been described as "life-savers" by many participants. If your community does not yet offer such training sessions, discuss this possibility with the medical or social service staff of the memory clinic you are attending, and encourage them to "go and do like-wise."

Driving

When should an Alzheimer's patient stop driving? This is a very important question. In our society our sense of independence is very much connected to being able to come and go as we please. In Alzheimer's disease, judgment and reaction speed may become impaired well before the straight-forward skills of operating an automobile become impaired. For this reason, patients with Alzheimer's disease should be persuaded fairly early on in the disease to trade off their own driving for being *chauffeur-driven* by their caregiver or by someone else. The risks of incurring an accident that may harm the patient or another person on the road, as well as the risk of financial loss due to an accident, are great indeed. When the patient with Alzheimer's disease cannot be persuaded to give up driving voluntarily, the patient's doctor should recommend to the patient and to the Bureau of Motor vehicles that the person not drive any more. If need be, you as a caregiver may want to disable the patient's automobile, openly or surreptitiously, so that the Alzheimer's patient will no longer be able to drive.

Eldercare Locator

The Eldercare Locator is a public service provided by the Administration on Aging of the US government. It provides a listing of all Area Agencies on Aging as well as all State Units on Aging. Through your local Area Agency on Aging you can find access to community health care, nutrition, home care, and caregiver services. Tel. 1-800-677-1116. Internet contact: Eldercare.gov.

Family history of Alzheimer's disease

Sometimes caregivers become concerned about the possibility that because someone else in their family has experienced Alzheimer's disease, they themselves are at greater risk for developing the disease. This concern is for the most part unwarranted. Advancing age is the greatest risk factor for developing Alzheimer's disease. For example, at age 65 only one percent of individuals have Alzheimer's. At age 75 this has risen to ten percent. At age 85 some 35 percent of such individuals have the disease, and at age 90, nearly fifty percent are affected by the disease. Having a single blood relative with Alzheimer's disease increased the risk for developing the disease only slightly. However, if both parents of an individual have had the disease, the risk for their offspring developing the disease increases substantially.

What I have tried to convey in this section is that hereditary factors do not play a major role in determining whether someone may be at risk for developing Alzheimer's disease *unless* two or more blood relatives have had the disease. On the other hand, some 0.5 percent of individuals suffer from a clearly inherited form of Alzheimer's disease. In these individuals the disease begins in the person's forties or fifties, and they generally do not survive much beyond their early sixties. In these individuals fully one half of all their offspring will inherit the disease.

Hospitalizations

Please be alert to the fact that hospitals have proven to be very inhospitable environments for patients with Alzheimer's disease. The relocation, the exposure to multiple strangers and strange procedures, the possibility of anesthesia or other medications added to the patient's usual medication regimen, have a definite deleterious effect on such patients. They are likely to become grossly disoriented, frightened, agitated, hostile, and delirious. Many such patients have begun to hallucinate or to become delusional shortly after admission, leading to responses from staff which makes their status even more precarious.

For this reason, hospitalization should be avoided, if at all possible, in favor of home care or continued care in a nursing home. However, when hospitalization is absolutely necessary, such as for instance for a hip fracture, the patient's principal caregiver should accompany the patient to the hospital, be in attendance or nearby at all times, and try to continue to re-orient the patient to their new setting, seeking to re-orient them over and over again. Attempts at sedation have often only made the situation worse, and restraints applied to the patient can be perfectly disastrous. In addition, it is important that for patients who have been on Alzheimer's medications, that these medications be restarted as quickly as possible. Alzheimer's medications are frequently discontinued when someone is admitted to a hospital.

Long-Distance Caregiving

Many caregivers are not located right at the site of where the patient is. In this situation I recommend that a local geriatric care manager be employed who can coordinate doctor visits, medication-taking, daycare or respite care, or eventual admission to a care facility. Just as the patient cannot report accurately on their memory problems or problems in living, neither will you be able to assess the problems long distance. Your local Alzheimer's Association chapter or Area Agency on Aging may be able to put you in touch with a geriatric care manager. An initial personal visit to where the patient lives is also recommended, with return visits as often as is feasible.

Long term care insurance

This type of insurance will provide for the cost of receiving long term care for a chronic illness that you or your spouse may need. Depending on the specific terms of your long term care insurance policy, this can include the cost of a nursing home, an assisted living facility or medical care that you receive in your home. The reason for insuring against long term care costs is that these can be very high indeed, and may continue over a period of months or even years. The cost of nursing home care may range anywhere from $60,000 to $120,000 per year, depending on where in the country this cost is incurred, with highest cost being experienced in the Northeast and California, with lowest cost in Southern states. Thus, over a period of several years, the cost of nursing home care can completely wipe out a considerable fortune.

The cost of long term care insurance can be very reasonable and affordable if it is purchased for an individual who is still relatively healthy. The cost for such insurance for someone who already has a condition which is likely to result in long term care, such as diabetes with complications, or Alzheimer's disease, is almost prohibitively expensive and often is not much less than the cost of paying for such care out of pocket. Moreover, once the disease has been diagnosed in an individual, it is unlikely that such a person will be granted this type of insurance. So it would be wise to acquire this type of insurance when the person covered is still free of any serious chronic disease.

The practical lesson to be learned from this discussion is that while it may be too late to acquire long-term care insurance for your loved affected with Alzheimer's disease, it may be just the right time to purchase such insurance for yourself while you are still in good health and while rates are still very reasonable for you.

Parkinson's disease

Parkinson's is a distinct and separate neurodegenerative disease that occurs with increasing frequency with advancing age. It is characterized by muscle tremors and stiff muscles, especially muscles of the face. These give the Parkinson's patient a typical mask-like face. There is an interesting reciprocal relationship between Parkinson's and Alzheimer's disease, as follows: Late in Parkinson's disease symptoms of dementia develop in perhaps fifteen percent of such patients. Similarly, late in Alzheimer's disease, Parkinsonian symptoms develop, again in perhaps fifteen percent of such patients. In addition, in a small number of individuals both diseases may occur simultaneously, which then worsen the overall disability experienced by the patient. In addition the progression of symptoms may be somewhat more rapid in patients who experience both diseases to their full extent.

Pervasive nihilism

Late in this disease there sometimes appears a pattern of behavior that is truly baffling and frustrating: the patient will say "no" to everything you propose, will refuse to do whatever you ask, and no amount of explaining or reasoning will change this. We can perhaps presume that the person is severely depressed, and is unwilling or unable to give any positive responses. I personally don't understand this phenomenon. Sometimes it goes away after a period of time. You might be able to hasten its disappearance by offering tender love and affection, accompanied by verbal reassurances or not. A trial of antidepressant medication may also be indicated. Perhaps someone in your support group will come up with an answer to this phenomenon. If you come across an answer, please let me know. I attribute it to an existential expression of the utter frustration that someone must feel over the fact that they have been afflicted with Alzheimer's disease.

Power of attorney

Patients in the early stages of Alzheimer's disease are still able to give valid power-of-attorney to the caregiver or another family member or outside advisor to act as the person's attorney. The requirements for this are very similar to those for making a will. Most patients with Alzheimer's should have someone who has power of attorney for them to make decisions on their behalf as they move further and further into this disease.

Seizures

A small proportion of patients with Alzheimer's disease may experience seizures solely as a result of the advancing Alzheimer's disease. If someone has seizures a medical workup for other causes of seizures, such as tumors or strokes, should be carried out. But if no other causes are found, the patient should be treated with anti-seizure medications such as the drug Dilantin or a similar drug prescribed to minimize the risk of recurrence of seizures.

Sex

The sexual behavior of patients with Alzheimer's disease is likely to change, along with other changes in their behavior. But there is no single pattern of such changes. In some patients interest in sex disappears, and while that may be regrettable, it is part and parcel of the general loss of interest experienced by many patients. It is by no means the worst problem for the caregiver to deal with. More troublesome may be two other types of changes in sexual behavior: an excessive preoccupation with sex and or excessively frequent demand for sex. Alternatively, the patient may be interested in having sex, but no longer remembers his or her own role and activities in performing sexual acts. It is advisable that you as a caregiver seek advice from your own physician, or else discuss the particular sexual problems you experience with your Alzheimer's patient's doctor. Also, other members in your support group will have faced similar issues, and they may have suggestions to offer to you as to how to cope with the problem.

Sleep Apnea

Sleep apnea is a phenomenon that can occur in patients with and without Alzheimer's disease. It is a cessation of respiration for perhaps several minutes, followed by deep, deep repeated respirations to get back into oxygen balance. Sleep characterized by sleep apnea is not as refreshing as regular sleep, and may make memory function even worse. In non-Alzheimer's patients a mask providing positive pressure oxygen can remedy the situation, but such a mask is generally poorly tolerated by Alzheimer's patients. The use of medications like Provigil or Nuvigil may reduce the frequency and the severity of sleep apnea.

"Smart Pills"

Any discussion of treating the symptoms of Alzheimer's disease quite naturally evokes a curiosity whether the medications used to treat Alzheimer's disease could also be used to prevent Alzheimer's disease, or whether they can be used by healthy individuals as "smart pills" to improve intellectual ability of normal or healthy individuals. At this time there are no solid data to support the use of these drugs either in an effort to prevent Alzheimer's disease, or to improve intellectual productivity. A few studies have shown some benefits of using these drugs in college students preparing for exams or in test pilots utilizing flight simulator machines. I would recommend waiting for further clarification of these issues before embarking on a course of just trying these medications on your own.

Undue influence

Undue influence is said to have occurred when a patient is "persuaded" to make a change in their will or other concession to benefit the caregiver under the threat that the patient will be placed in a nursing home or otherwise will no longer be cared for by the specific caregiver. Proof of such undue influences will invalidate any such change or provision in a will. It is generally viewed as a situation in which a weakened mind is influenced to make a decision favorable to the caregiver, under duress.

Weight loss

When weight loss begins to occur in a patient with advanced Alzheimer's disease, in the absence of any other specific disease, such as a gastrointestinal problem or cancer, it should be a warning sign that the end may be approaching. At this point the patient should be encouraged to eat frequent meals with high fat or calorie count, such as ice-cream, peanut butter, or fried foods which the patient can enjoy, without worrying about cholesterol levels or diabetes. Maintenance of weight will be beneficial, but in general no heroic measures, such a tube feeding or intravenous feedings, are indicated.

About the Author:

Dr. Eric Pfeiffer is a nationally and internationally recognized authority on health and aging. He is the Founding Director of the Suncoast Alzheimer's and Gerontology Center at the University of South Florida College of Medicine. He is the author of several major textbooks on health and aging, including *Behavior and Adaptation in Late Life* and *Mental Illness in Late Life,* both published by Little, Brown. He is now retired from medical practice and is devoting his time to writing and speaking to lay and professional audiences about successful aging and about caregiving in Alzheimer's disease.

In 1977 Dr. Pfeiffer was awarded the Allen Gold Medal for outstanding achievement in the area of Geriatric Psychiatry by the American Geriatric society. In 1985 Dr. Pfeiffer was honored for his work in the area of Alzheimer's disease through the establishment of the Eric Pfeiffer Chair in Alzheimer's disease Research at the University of South Florida. Most recently, Dr. Pfeiffer has been nominated for the Senior Living Media Award of the Florida Council on Aging, largely on the basis of his two most recent books, "14 Winning Strategies for Successful Aging" and "The Art of Caregiving in Alzheimer's Disease."

Dr. Pfeiffer has conducted numerous studies on new medications for use with Alzheimer's patients and individuals with minor cognitive impairment. These studies include work with each of the cholinesterase inhibitors, Aricept, Exelon and Razadyne, as well as with Namenda.

Dr. Pfeiffer has published widely in many scientific journals on topics related to health, mental health, and aging. He has lectured at many universities, colleges and professional organizations.

Dr. Pfeiffer is also a published poet. His book, "Take with Me Now That Enormous Step" was winner of the Charioteer Poetry Award. His second book of Poems, entitled "Under One Roof" has just been published. Some of his poems have appeared in JAMA and in The Pharos.